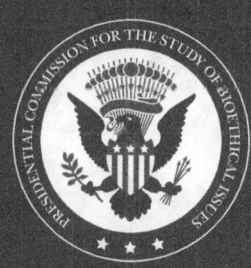

BIOETHICS FOR EVERY GENERATION

Deliberation and Education in Health, Science, and Technology

Presidential Commission
for the Study of Bioethical Issues

May 2016

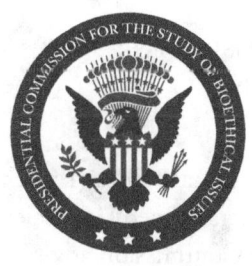

BIOETHICS FOR EVERY GENERATION
Deliberation and Education in Health, Science, and Technology

Presidential Commission
for the **Study of Bioethical Issues**

Washington, D.C.
May 2016

http://www.bioethics.gov

ABOUT THE PRESIDENTIAL COMMISSION FOR
THE STUDY OF BIOETHICAL ISSUES

The Presidential Commission for the Study of Bioethical Issues (Bioethics Commission) is an advisory panel of the nation's leaders in medicine, science, ethics, religion, law, and engineering. The Bioethics Commission advises the President on bioethical issues arising from advances in biomedicine and related areas of science and technology. The Bioethics Commission seeks to identify and promote policies and practices that ensure scientific research, health care delivery, and technological innovation are conducted in a socially and ethically responsible manner.

For more information about the Bioethics Commission, please see http://www.bioethics.gov.

The use of trade names and commercial sources in this report is for identification only and does not imply endorsement.

CONTENTS

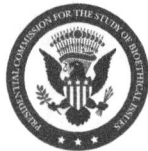

PRESIDENTIAL COMMISSION FOR THE STUDY OF BIOETHICAL ISSUES

President Barack Obama
The White House
1600 Pennsylvania Avenue, NW
Washington, DC 20500

Dear Mr. President:

On behalf of the Presidential Commission for the Study of Bioethical Issues (Bioethics Commission), we present to you *Bioethics for Every Generation: Deliberation and Education in Health, Science, and Technology*. In this legacy report, the Bioethics Commission focuses on two essential, mutually reinforcing missions—both practical and ethical—in our constitutional democracy: democratic deliberation and ethics education. These two tools can and should be used in tandem to address and resolve complex problems in developing health, science, and technology policy for our society.

A primary mission of the Bioethics Commission has been to reimagine and reinvigorate the deliberative and educational roles of bioethics commissions in our democracy. Expanding the reach of our many in-person meetings, we have used online media tools for public outreach and input, and we have developed an unprecedented range of educational materials that help tailor our work to a variety of audiences. We undertook this report—which focuses on the future of bioethics deliberation and education—because of our nation's urgent ongoing need to foster civil and robust public discourse and civic involvement, especially in service of health, science, and technology policy that serves the common good.

The Bioethics Commission approached each of its past projects with robust and reasoned deliberation, inviting presentations from a variety of experts and leaders, soliciting and receiving thoughtful input from the public, and conducting almost 200 hours of public discussion over seven years. In each

1425 NEW YORK AVENUE, NW, SUITE C-100, WASHINGTON, DC 20005
PHONE 202-233-3960 FAX 202-233-3990 WWW.BIOETHICS.GOV

of its reports, the Bioethics Commission has recommended improvements in ethics and bioethics education. The Bioethics Commission's body of over 60 accompanying educational materials is already aiding in the integration of bioethics into classrooms and professional settings across our country, from high schools to hospitals and beyond. These educational materials reflect the Bioethics Commission's commitment to develop useful and accessible tools that enable and encourage all citizens to familiarize themselves with the most important developments in health, science, and technology.

To inform this capstone report, the Bioethics Commission held four public meetings with deliberation and education as the focus, and heard from speakers with diverse backgrounds and perspectives. The Bioethics Commission also received many thoughtful public comments.

In *Bioethics for Every Generation*, the Bioethics Commission offers eight recommendations to increase and improve the use of democratic deliberation and ethics education in order to enhance complex decision making in bioethics and health, science, and technology policy at all levels. Because education and deliberation are mutually reinforcing, we offer ideas for innovative ways to incorporate deliberation skills into ethics education, and to enhance deliberative processes by improving ethics education.

The Bioethics Commission is honored by the trust you have placed in us and appreciative of the opportunity to serve you and our nation in this way.

Sincerely,

Amy Gutmann, Ph.D.
Chair

James W. Wagner, Ph.D.
Vice Chair

PRESIDENTIAL COMMISSION FOR THE STUDY OF BIOETHICAL ISSUES

AMY GUTMANN, Ph.D., CHAIR
President and Christopher H. Browne
Distinguished Professor of Political Science and Professor of Communication,
University of Pennsylvania

JAMES W. WAGNER, Ph.D., VICE CHAIR
President, Emory University

ANITA L. ALLEN, J.D., Ph.D.
Vice Provost for Faculty,
Henry R. Silverman Professor of Law
and Professor of Philosophy,
University of Pennsylvania

BARBARA F. ATKINSON, M.D.
Founding Dean,
University of Nevada, Las Vegas
School of Medicine

NITA A. FARAHANY, J.D., Ph.D.
Director, Duke Initiative for
Science & Society;
Director, Duke M.A. in Bioethics and
Science Policy, Professor of Law and
Philosophy, Duke University

CHRISTINE GRADY, R.N., Ph.D.
Chief, Department of Bioethics,
National Institutes of Health
Clinical Center

STEPHEN L. HAUSER, M.D.
Director, UCSF Weill Institute for
Neurosciences; Robert A. Fishman
Distinguished Professor and Chair
of the Department of Neurology,
University of California, San Francisco

RAJU S. KUCHERLAPATI, Ph.D.
Paul C. Cabot Professor, Department
of Genetics, Harvard Medical School;
Professor, Department of Medicine,
Brigham and Women's Hospital

NELSON L. MICHAEL, M.D., Ph.D.
Colonel, Medical Corps, U.S. Army;
Director, U.S. Military HIV Research
Program, Walter Reed Army Institute
of Research

DANIEL P. SULMASY, M.D., Ph.D., FACP
Kilbride-Clinton Professor of Medicine
and Ethics, Department of Medicine
and Divinity School; Associate Director,
The MacLean Center for Clinical Medical
Ethics, University of Chicago

*Former Members**

YOLANDA ALI
Michael J. Fox Foundation
Founders' Council;
Emory Neurosciences
Community Advisory Board

JOHN D. ARRAS, Ph.D.
Porterfield Professor of Biomedical
Ethics; Professor of Philosophy;
Professor of Public Health Sciences;
University of Virginia

ALEXANDER G. GARZA, M.D., M.P.H.
Assistant Secretary, Office of Health
Affairs; Chief Medical Officer,
Department of Homeland Security

*Affiliation at time of Commission membership.
*John D. Arras was a member of the Presidential Commission for the Study of Bioethical Issues from May 2010
until his death in March 2015. The Bioethics Commission recognizes his contributions to its ongoing reflections on
education during this time, informed by his over 46 years of experience in teaching.*

PRESIDENTIAL COMMISSION FOR THE STUDY OF BIOETHICAL ISSUES

STAFF AND CONSULTANTS

Executive Director
Lisa M. Lee, Ph.D., M.A., M.S.

Associate Director
Kata Chillag, Ph.D.

Senior Advisors
Paul A. Lombardo, Ph.D., J.D.
Jonathan D. Moreno, Ph.D.

Research Staff, Fellows, and Interns*
James Aluri, M.A.
Misti Ault Anderson, M.S., M.A.
Elizabeth M. Fenton, Ph.D., M.P.H.
Perry Goffner
Steven Kessler, M.S.
Karen M. Meagher, Ph.D.
Michael Moorin
Cristina Nigro, M.S.
Elizabeth R. Pike, J.D., LL.M.
Maneesha Sakhuja, M.H.S.
Nicolle K. Strand, J.D., M. Bioethics
Victoria Wilbur, B.A.
Tenny R. Zhang, B.A.

Administrative Staff
Tynetta Dreher
Esther E. Yoo

Consultants
Bonnie Hamalainen, M.F.A
Burness Communications
C. Kay Smith, M.Ed.

*Includes former research staff, fellows, and interns

ACKNOWLEDGEMENTS

This report reflects the culmination of our nearly eight years of work as the Presidential Commission for the Study of Bioethical Issues. We are grateful to our former members, Lonnie Ali, Alex Garza, and John Arras whose contributions to our deliberations reflect a deep and abiding dedication to public service and learning.

We are grateful to each of the over 200 speakers who provided us with personal and professional testimony that enabled us to consider a breadth of perspectives on disparate topics over the years. We appreciate their candor, their clarity, and their engagement with the important issues placed before us. In addition, we appreciate the hundreds of public comments we received on the various topics that we addressed; this public participation in bioethical issues was essential for us to arrive at legitimate recommendations.

We are indebted to our capable and committed staff whose energy, careful research, and variety of expertise made indelible contributions to our success. Executive Director Lisa M. Lee and senior advisors Paul A. Lombardo and Jonathan D. Moreno led and inspired staff to do their best work, which allowed us to meet the numerous complex demands we faced. Valerie H. Bonham, who served as Executive Director during our first two years, was instrumental in getting us off to a productive start. Associate Directors Michelle Groman and Kayte Spector-Bagdady, and later Kata Chillag, provided impeccable logistic and production support for our reports in addition to subject matter expertise. Communications Director Hillary Wicai Viers and Communications Assistant Alannah Kittle ensured that our activities and materials reached the right audience at their release and laid the path for their enduring use. We thank the following staff members and advisors for their contributions across the Bioethics Commission's tenure:

Anne Pierson Allen
Misti Ault Anderson
Kavita M. Berger
Rachel S. Bressler
David DeGrazia
Brian C. Eiler
Elizabeth M. Fenton

Debbie Forrest
Holly Fernandez Lynch
Eleanor E. Mayer
Debra J.H. Mathews
Karen M. Meagher
David G. Miller
Cristina Nigro

Elizabeth R. Pike
Alan Rubel
Maneesha Sakhuja
Cary Scheiderer
Nicolle K. Strand
Jason L. Schwartz
Jeremy Sugarman

Bonnie Hamalainen of NIH Division of Medical Arts provided expert design advice and service across the body of our work. Tynetta Dreher and Esther Yoo served as the administrative glue, consistently going above and beyond to ensure Bioethics Commission members and our guest speakers were able to gather around the same table to deliberate. To the many Research Associates, fellows, interns, and others with whom we have had the pleasure of working, we thank you.

For their contributions to *Bioethics for Every Generation*, we are grateful to the 23 presenters who spoke before the Bioethics Commission about deliberation and ethics education. We also acknowledge that this report is informed and enriched by the many other speakers who have commented on deliberation and ethics education over the years while presenting to the Bioethics Commission on topics addressed in previous reports. We would like to recognize and thank our staff for expert assistance in completing this report, as well. A special thanks to *Bioethics for Every Generation*'s project lead Elizabeth Fenton and to Nicolle K. Strand for expert drafting of the volume.

Our deepest appreciation goes to Executive Director Lisa M. Lee and Senior Policy and Research Analyst Misti Ault Anderson for envisioning a substantial role for us in the bioethics education landscape. Their steadfast commitment to and expertise in bioethics education has served us well.

EXECUTIVE SUMMARY

Bioethics permeates multiple facets of our public and private lives. The Presidential Commission for the Study of Bioethical Issues (Bioethics Commission) has tackled challenges that all of us face as individuals, professionals, family members, and members of society in an increasingly interconnected world. Such questions include, among others, whether and how to employ advancing technology, how researchers and health care providers should behave in certain situations, how governments should handle public health emergencies, and how individuals should incorporate their values when making decisions on behalf of loved ones. Taken together, these questions get to the heart of what it means to be a participant in our democracy and, in an even broader sense, a responsible member of our world. Tackling these questions requires careful and reasoned deliberation, as well as a comprehensive understanding of the values that each of us brings to the discussion. Deliberation and education are joined in a virtuous circle, reinforcing one another to create a more democratic and just society.

Addressing these important questions, which have both practical and ethical dimensions, requires a thoughtful deliberative process, because disagreement is not something that individuals, professionals, or public officials can or should avoid.[1] Arriving at publicly defensible answers to these questions requires careful and reasoned deliberation as well as a comprehensive understanding of the values that each of us brings to the discussion. The range of relevant values—whether part of an individual's ethics or a professional's obligations—can be in conflict, and those value conflicts require reconciliation and sometimes public negotiation. For example, in health and science policy, we often must address the tension between the importance of individual autonomy on one side of the debate and the potential for great societal benefit on the other. We must consider how to protect against risk while also advancing science and finding cures for diseases or injury-prevention strategies. In modeling a process for addressing these questions and steering a way forward, the Bioethics Commission has demonstrated that democratic deliberation and ethics education complement one another, raising the level of discourse about difficult bioethical concerns and improving the way we address ethical challenges in health, science, and technology.

The first part of this report provides a justification for the value and use of democratic deliberation in bioethics, sets forth a roadmap for conducting democratic deliberation, and outlines recommendations for advancing and improving its use in solving complex bioethics and health policy problems. Democratic deliberation about these problems requires an understanding of their ethical dimensions. This ethical understanding develops in large part through education in ethics. Ethics education provides stakeholders with the tools for understanding, reasoning through, and articulating their own values when making good decisions about bioethics and health for themselves, their loved ones, or their communities and society.

The second part of this report explores possibilities for building on the Bioethics Commission's past work on education by recommending the infusion of bioethics training throughout education, building knowledge and skills that are tailored for different educational levels and life stages. Even as young children are beginning school, they can grasp general ethics concepts such as right and wrong. As older students focus their interests and begin work or professional training, ethics education can and should become more topic-specific. This report outlines recommendations for how ethics education can be enhanced at all stages and in different educational contexts with the goal of increasing ethical readiness for engagement in civil deliberation about bioethical concerns.

Ethics education is crucial for robust democratic deliberation, and deliberation broadens participants' interest in and understanding of different perspectives and values that exist in their communities.[2] Deliberation and education complement one another, elevating the level of discourse and improving the way our society resolves morally complex challenges in health, science, and technology. This report concludes by recommending a path to strengthen the association between deliberation and education and to ensure that both are reflected in the work of future bioethics advisory bodies and in society more broadly.

Democratic Deliberation in Bioethics

Democratic deliberation is a method of decision making in which participants discuss and debate a question of common concern, justifying their arguments with reasons and treating one another with mutual respect, with the goal of reaching an actionable decision for policy or law, open to future challenge or revision.[3] The process of democratic deliberation is especially useful for the types of ethical questions we face in bioethics, in which solutions have complex empirical as well as moral bases and about which reasonable people can disagree. Bioethics advisory bodies can play a key role in leading these deliberations on the local, state, national, and international levels.

Effective democratic deliberation calls for inclusive and respectful debate and depends on collaborative decision making. Stakeholders with a range of perspectives are encouraged to present their views, seek common ground whenever possible, and maintain mutual respect even when irreconcilable differences among viewpoints remain.[4]

The notion of collaborative decision making and inclusion of a range of perspectives is especially important when deliberating about bioethics. Bioethics is inherently interdisciplinary and involves questions of broad public concern that can be technical and complicated, both scientifically and ethically. Effective deliberation about these topics requires careful presentation and analysis of information as well as inclusion of all relevant viewpoints and stakeholders, from scientists and health care providers who are experts in the technology or policy being deliberated, to members of the public who will be affected by a decision, to professionals across a diversity of fields who can understand the implications of a policy for the law, industry, government, and beyond.

The field of bioethics is often called upon to resolve seemingly intractable ethical conflicts and challenges.[5] Distributing scarce health resources, determining which patient should receive an organ available for transplant, or determining when restricting individuals' liberty for the community's safety and wellbeing is justifiable are central questions in bioethics that cannot be resolved except through a process in which multiple perspectives are shared and considered. These debates occur at all governmental levels in addition to communities, hospitals, institutional review boards, and professional societies. Deliberation is an essential process for finding points of agreement and moving forward on these morally complex concerns in all of these contexts.

Recommendation 1: Guide Bioethics Policy Decisions with Democratic Deliberation

Stakeholders in the democratic process at all levels—including communities, policymakers, popular opinion leaders, and advisory bodies—should use a

well-crafted form of democratic deliberation to inform and guide health, science, and technology policy decisions and their ethical dimensions. Policymakers, communities, and advisory bodies should use democratic deliberation to consider morally complex and controversial bioethical problems to promote mutual understanding and respect among participants as well as greater legitimacy for resulting policy.

Successful democratic deliberation fosters greater individual and mutual understanding of problems of common concern, broader public engagement with complex policy questions, and legitimacy of decision making. Both immediate and long-term benefits result from diverse stakeholders in our democracy participating in forums for decision making that reflect the core values of democratic deliberation.[6]

Recommendation 2: Conduct Deliberative Activities in Ways Conducive to Mutual Respect and Reason-Giving Among Participants in Accordance with Best Practices

Organizers of deliberative activities should ensure that deliberation is accomplished in accordance with best practices established in the broad body of scholarly literature. At a minimum, effective deliberative processes require participants to give reasons for their arguments and to show respect for fellow participants. In addition, the set of concerns for deliberation should raise questions for which practical decisions need to be made, and the deliberations should be intended and designed to influence how those decisions are made.

Individuals and entities that organize deliberative processes, or would like to incorporate democratic deliberation into their decision-making processes, should review and incorporate existing literature on methods and best practices. Steps in the process are described below and are included in Appendix I (Steps for Deliberation). Other considerations include how long to deliberate, how many individuals to include, whether to seek a random sample or ensure inclusion from members of certain groups, what preparatory materials to make available, and how to incorporate expert consultation and supply useful information for those engaged in deliberation. Regardless of variations in the deliberative process, at a minimum, it should require that participants give reasons for their views and show respect for one another.

As a concrete demonstration of respect, decisions should aim, if possible, to enable minority practices to continue to flourish, provided these practices do not threaten the common good or unduly burden the majority's ability to implement the agreed-upon policy. Additional best practices will depend on the particular goals and context of the deliberative activity.

Recommendation 3: To Further the Practical Contribution of Deliberation in Bioethics, Conduct Additional Research on the Effectiveness of Deliberative Methods

Scholars of democratic deliberation, along with individuals and organizations using democratic deliberation for decision making, should continue to assess the effectiveness of particular deliberative methods as tools to address complex bioethical challenges. These studies should evaluate the processes and outcomes of different kinds of deliberation and establish measurements of success.

During the past decade, scholars have begun to develop and refine measures for evaluating the effectiveness of deliberative activities.[7] In evaluating these activities, they have been attentive to both processes and outcomes, but more work remains. Specifically, formative and process evaluations should include questions about how to conduct democratic deliberation to maximize mutual respect, optimize engagement, and elicit less commonly held perspectives to create an inclusive discussion of policy proposals. Public health policies are a particularly important area for public deliberation because they require cooperation among substantial portions of the population. A deliberative approach that engages affected communities and uses deliberative processes to reach policy solutions that are both ethically and scientifically sound leads to public health policies with greater legitimacy for those most affected by them.

Bioethics Education

Regardless of whether we are aware of it, bioethics affects us all. As individuals, we have no alternative but to navigate an increasingly complex health care system for ourselves and our loved ones. As voters, taxpayers, and community members, we must decide what communal values should guide policy on fundamental questions of birth and death, health, and wellbeing—or these will be decided for us. As scientists, clinicians, and lawyers, to fulfill our professional obligations, we must resolve dilemmas, understand the obligations of our professions, and attend to the broader social impacts of our work. In each of these roles, the ability to recognize, articulate, and resolve ethical challenges is absolutely essential.

National bioethics bodies like ours can accept an increasingly important role by encouraging and supporting bioethics education. This Bioethics Commission has strived to fulfill this role in several ways. We have developed educational materials related to our reports to reach diverse audiences. We participate in deliberation and learn details of particular topics to gain a deeper understanding of how ethics principles we have learned throughout our lives, both personally and professionally, should be applied to the open questions we face as a federal commission. In modeling this educational component of deliberative democracy, we aim to encourage future generations of bioethicists, scientists, health care providers, other professionals, and the public at large to become informed and make reasoned decisions in this pluralistic society. As the Bioethics Commission nears the end of its tenure, we encourage future bioethics advisory bodies to continue to fulfill this role, as bodies before us have done.

Ethics education should start early, building a foundation for ongoing learning throughout education. Early ethics education provides a base on which to build skills to engage with the ethical dimensions of subjects taught in postsecondary school, as well as ethical matters in specific professions. In addition, ethics education at different stages of life helps individuals grapple with ethical choices as individuals, family and community members, and professionals.

Ethics education can and should be incorporated throughout education, from curricula in primary school through secondary school, to undergraduate coursework, graduate school, and professional training programs. Ethics education is best when it builds on itself over time. To build ethics literacy, broad-based ethics education must start early, before students begin to track into more specialized interests and careers. Over time, ethics education should become more targeted, and provide preparation for the particular challenges that health, science, and technology professionals are likely to face.

Recommendation 4: Implement Foundational Broad-Based Ethics Education at all Levels

Educators at all levels, from preschool to postsecondary and professional schools, should integrate ethics education across the curriculum to prepare students for engaging with morally complex questions in a diverse range of subjects. Ethics education should include attention to both the development of moral character and virtue as well as the cultivation of ethical reasoning and decision-making skills that can be deployed in a bioethics context. Methods of ethics education should be evidence-based and grounded in best practices.

Development of ethical reasoning skills begins early in childhood. Questions and case studies with a bioethical component can be an important element of this early education. For example, elementary school students might be asked to think about what questions they would have if they were invited to participate in research. Older elementary school students might be asked to compare theories arrived at by science versus those arrived at by other methods or to reason through the concept of neurobiologic determinism by answering such discussion questions as, "Are our futures and fates fixed? Does what we do today have any effect on what happens in the future?"[8] Ethics education builds critical thinking and argumentation skills, develops character, and emphasizes the importance of virtue. Those who develop curricula should draw from the empirical evidence about moral development to scaffold questions and topics that are tailored for students' level of thinking at different ages.[9]

Recommendation 5: Develop Bioethics Education and Training for Professionals

Educators at the graduate and professional levels, including in the health care, public health, engineering, and legal fields, should develop, integrate, and emphasize bioethics education to foster continued character development, cultivate a culture of responsibility, and teach the specific skills and bioethical reasoning applicable to the profession.

Professional ethics seeks to identify and guide professionals' actions on the basis of the moral foundations of their chosen careers, and these actions often need to be explicitly taught. Graduate programs in such professions as nursing and public health ought to help students develop the confidence, reasoning skills, and moral resources they will need to address the distinct ethical considerations of their professional work. Importantly, some graduate programs including laboratory science and public health have independently documented a need to develop critical reasoning skills and moral sensitivity.[10]

Recommendation 6: Support Opportunities for Teacher Training in Bioethics Education

Education policymakers, teacher training programs, and other funders should support development of teacher training in ethics education to prepare teachers of all subjects to facilitate constructive bioethical conversations in their classrooms. Teacher training programs should anticipate existing educational inequities and provide teachers and students with equitable access to ethics education, with an aim of preparing all students for the bioethical questions that might arise during the course of their lives.

Educators need support and professional development that prepares them to overcome obstacles to implementing bioethics education and that rewards them for doing so. Training in ethics and techniques for conducting deliberative discussions in the classroom can help teachers overcome their own and others' hesitancy to engage in bioethics education. Training also can prepare teachers for addressing administrators' and parents' concerns that ethics education seeks to indoctrinate students.

Mutual Reinforcement of Deliberation and Ethics Education

Ethics education, through its focus on engagement with values and analytical reasoning, prepares members of communities to engage with and deliberate about morally complex bioethical questions arising in science and technology. In turn, deliberative practices are educational, leading to a more informed and participatory public. These mutually reinforcing functions create a virtuous circle, reflecting the ways in which ethics education and democratic deliberation are linked. Learning to recognize, articulate, and resolve the different ethical challenges we encounter as individuals will foster the skills necessary for deliberating with others about contentious civic concerns we face in our increasingly pluralistic society. In other words, education is crucially important for democratic citizenship.[11] Deliberation can be used as a tool to develop more informed and educated students, professionals, communities, and leaders who can constructively contribute to conversations about morally complex topics—including bioethical ones. The mutual reinforcement of deliberation and ethics education promotes values essential to an engaged and civic-minded population.

Recommendation 7: Foster Mutual Reinforcement of Deliberation and Ethics Education

Educators and organizers of deliberative activities should use the tools of deliberation and education to facilitate civic engagement about pressing bioethical concerns surrounding developments in health, science, and technology.

This Bioethics Commission has demonstrated its commitment to furthering ethics education at all levels, by making recommendations calling for both broad public ethics education and specific professional ethics training, as well as developing bioethics educational materials that can be used in a broad range of settings by educators who want to incorporate bioethics into their classrooms. The Bioethics Commission has developed more than 60 educational tools at the time of this printing and is continuing to develop more, including case studies, deliberation exercises, modules on key bioethics topics, classroom discussion guides, videos, and webinars, all of which are available for free download on the Commission's website. The materials can be used by teachers in high school, college, and graduate school classes; by professionals in the health sciences and technology fields, including clinicians, public health practitioners, and researchers; and by members of the public.

Recommendation 8: Encourage Future Bioethics Commissions to Further Their Deliberative and Educational Roles

Future bioethics commissions should continue to explore, reimagine, and reinvigorate the educational and democratic roles fulfilled and exemplified by such commissions. They also should encourage discourse and civic involvement in developing health, science, and technology policy. The work of bioethics commissions should be used as the foundation for creating educational tools tailored for different levels, from primary school through postgraduate and professional training, that enable teachers to introduce deliberation about contemporary and meaningful bioethics topics in their classrooms.

Supporting public bioethics education and engaging in deliberation are important functions of bioethics advisory bodies. Bioethics commissions ought to serve as public forums by engaging, educating, and listening and responding to citizens.[12] This Bioethics Commission has actively engaged in and helped to implement deliberative practices and bioethics education. It has made direct contributions to bioethics education by developing teaching tools that are wide-ranging in scope and format and intended to be accessible to both educators and members of the public. These materials draw on research about effective education to ensure that all kinds of learners are able to access the work of the Bioethics Commission, and through that work, engage in some of the most challenging contemporary bioethics topics.

* * *

Since its inception, this Bioethics Commission has been committed to the values embedded in democratic deliberation. We hope that this report informs, inspires, and guides future bioethics commissions. We have described our deliberative processes, outlining the key steps in the process of democratic deliberation, and recommended ways of incorporating and extending a deliberation approach to making recommendations and formulating advice on complex ethical challenges in health, science, and technology. As the tenure of this Bioethics Commission draws to a close, we hope that future commissions and advisory bodies at all levels will continue to invoke the values of democratic deliberation as they work to find ways forward on the most pressing bioethical questions that confront our society.

CHAPTER 1
Introduction

Democracy has to be born anew every generation,
and education is its midwife.[13]

—John Dewey, American educator and philosopher, 1859–1952

In the late 1980s, the state of Oregon attempted to pass a new budget that, in part, would reduce the cost of health care. The proposed budget cut coverage for common but expensive medical procedures from the state's publicly funded health care plan, drawing widespread public outcry.[14] Oregon state officials quickly discovered that such major decisions about government health care benefits should not be imposed on the public unilaterally. These decisions, which affect everyone, arouse deeply held values about what government owes its citizens and what citizens owe one another. They are best vetted through a consultative public process. The legitimacy of government action, more often than not, depends on inclusion of the governed in the decision-making process.

The Oregon case is particularly instructive. A deliberative process involving the public was needed—and eventually implemented—to create a prioritized list of health benefits that citizens viewed as legitimate. Legislative decisions about rationing health care, as with many policy decisions related to health and wellbeing, are value-laden and have profound consequences for all. As this report will demonstrate, democratic deliberation dramatically increases the likelihood that health policies will be accepted as legitimate and justifiable. It expresses due respect for those who will be governed by such policies.

The Presidential Commission for the Study of Bioethical Issues (Bioethics Commission) focuses on bioethics, which raises a diverse set of complex and weighty questions that will challenge nearly all of us at some point in our lives, as individuals and as members of our communities. A sample of the challenges this Commission has tackled include the following: How should we safeguard children from potential bioterrorism while ensuring their safety as we test medical countermeasures? What should doctors, researchers, and online health care companies do when they find something they did not expect (e.g., information indicating that an individual might develop an incurable disease)? How should the United States and other countries participate in global efforts to curtail outbreaks of highly infectious diseases such as the Ebola virus without compromising the liberty of their residents, mistreating aid workers, or contributing to the stigmatization of affected groups? How can we move forward with promising large-scale genomic research while protecting individual privacy? What are the implications of using new and innovative neuroscience research and technology to make us smarter or as evidence in a court of law?

Considering bioethical questions is at the heart of what it means to be an active participant in our democracy—whether as a clinician caring for patients, a family member making decisions for an ill relative, a company making personalized medical data available to consumers, a policymaker deciding how to regulate research, or a scientist advancing important discoveries. Addressing these important considerations, which have both practical and ethical dimensions, requires a thoughtful deliberative process, because disagreement is not something that individuals, professionals, or public officials can or should avoid.[15] Arriving at publicly defensible answers to each of these questions requires careful and reasoned deliberation as well as a comprehensive understanding of the values that each of us brings to the discussion.

The range of relevant values—whether part of an individual's ethics or a professional's obligations—can be in conflict, and those value conflicts require reconciliation and sometimes public negotiation. For example, in health and science policy, we often must address the tensions between the importance of individual autonomy on one side of the debate and the potential for great societal benefit on the other. In another example, we must consider how to protect against risk while also advancing science and finding cures for diseases or injury-prevention strategies. In modeling a process for addressing these questions and steering a way forward, the Bioethics Commission has demonstrated that democratic deliberation and ethics education complement one another, raising the level of discourse about difficult bioethical concerns and improving the way we address ethical challenges in health, science, and technology.

Respect, compromise, and constructive public engagement are values embedded in the theory and practice of democratic deliberation. Democratic deliberation is an essential tool for building constructive policy and practices, especially in a climate of polarization and distrust regarding government and public officials.

Democratic deliberation is a decision-making process in which participants give reasons for their views and decisions and respond to the reasons given by others in return. Reason-giving ensures that decisions made are justifiable and reflects the value of mutual respect for those who might be bound by such decisions, treating them as individuals who participate in their own governance.

The first part of this report provides a justification for the value and use of democratic deliberation in bioethics, sets forth a roadmap for conducting democratic deliberation, and outlines recommendations for advancing and improving its use in solving complex bioethics and health policy problems. Democratic deliberation about these problems requires an understanding of their ethical dimensions. This ethical understanding develops in large part through education in ethics. Ethics education provides stakeholders with the tools for understanding, reasoning through, and articulating their own values when making good decisions about bioethics and health for themselves, their loved ones, or their communities and society.

The Bioethics Commission also has prioritized bioethics education—both through its own public deliberation and in its published work. In its reports, the Bioethics Commission has confronted almost a dozen distinct bioethics topics—each one involves technical and scientific information and a set of values that are understood and weighed differently in each case. Throughout the course of its tenure, Commission members have addressed these topics methodically, always beginning by developing a thorough understanding of the scientific and ethical principles at stake. In this way, the Bioethics Commission has attempted to model effective ethics education as a fundamental element of deliberating and reaching agreeable recommendations and solutions at the federal policy level. In addition, the Bioethics Commission has produced more than 60 diverse educational materials, designed for audiences of different levels and disciplines from high school students to clinicians, lawyers, and other professionals. In each of its reports, the Commission has emphasized the importance of education for all members of society with a stake in the topic, because education helps raise the level of public discourse and contributes to more robust and legitimate policy decisions about these complex bioethics questions.

The second part of this report explores possibilities for building on the Bioethics Commission's past work on education by recommending the infusion of bioethics training throughout education, building knowledge and skills at different educational levels and life stages. Even as young children begin school, they can grasp such general ethics concepts as right and wrong. As older students focus their interests and begin work or professional training, ethics education can and should become more topic-specific. This report outlines recommendations for how ethics education can be enhanced at all stages and in different educational contexts with the goal of increasing ethical readiness for engagement in civil deliberation about bioethical concerns.

Ethics education is important for individuals making decisions that involve bioethics on a personal level—decisions about how aggressively to treat a terminal illness, whether to participate in medical research, or whether to use an emerging scientific technology—and can help individuals recognize ethical challenges while reflecting on the values implicit in them. Individuals also confront bioethics in decisions about policies and laws that will affect them and their neighbors—questions about who should be covered by publicly funded health care, whether physician-assisted dying should be available for individuals with terminal illness, or whether and how the public health department ought to nudge the public toward habits that might improve health and wellness or prevent obesity. Ethics education can help prepare individuals to deliberate and decide together what these policies should be and what values they should reflect.

Deliberation and education are joined
in a virtuous circle, reinforcing one another to create
a more democratic and just society.

Ethics education is crucial for robust democratic deliberation, and deliberation broadens participants' interest in and understanding of different perspectives and values that exist in their communities.[16] Deliberation and education are joined in a virtuous circle, reinforcing one another to create a more democratic and just society. This report concludes by recommending a path to strengthen the association between deliberation and education and to ensure that both are reflected in the work of future bioethics advisory bodies and in society more broadly.

About This Report

Throughout its tenure, the Bioethics Commission has completed 10 projects, including this one, on topics as diverse as privacy and whole genome sequencing, ethics and Ebola virus disease, and neuroscience and society (Figure 1). Presented with topics that involve deeply held values, public concern, and longstanding bioethical questions, the Bioethics Commission has approached each project with reasoned deliberation. They have invited testimony from experts in various disciplines and from across the country and the world, solicited input from the public, and conducted approximately 200 hours of public discussion over 7 years. Deliberation has been a key feature of this Bioethics Commission's work.

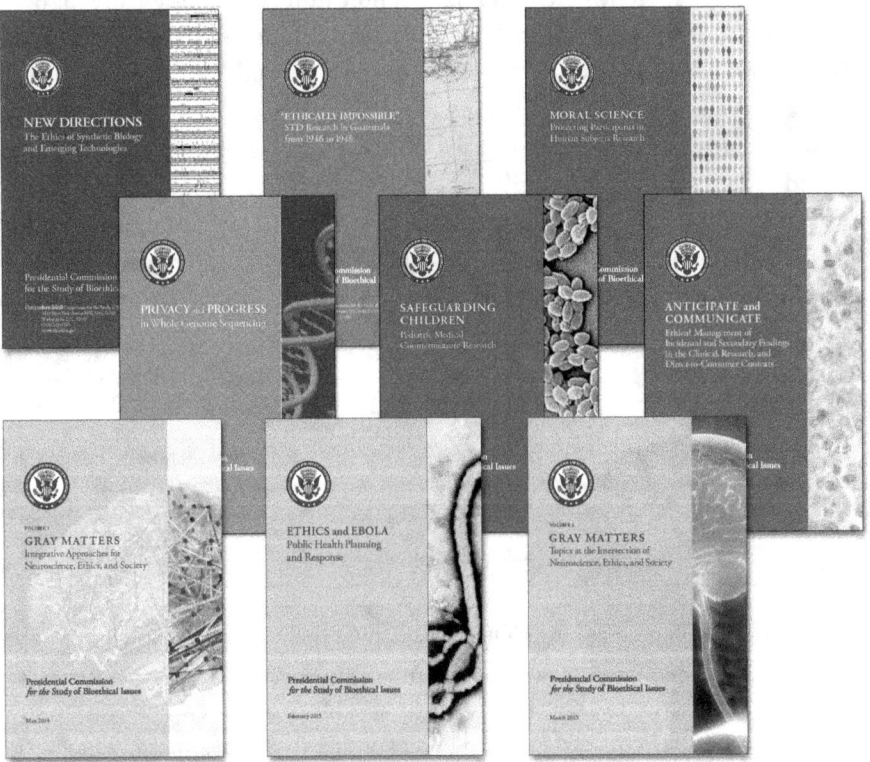

FIGURE 1: THE BIOETHICS COMMISSION'S REPORTS, 2010–2015

Since its inception in 2010, the Bioethics Commission has published nine reports, not including this one. Topics include synthetic biology, protection of human research participants, public health planning and response, and neuroscience, among others.

In each of its reports, the Bioethics Commission's substantive recommendations have included improvements in ethics and bioethics education to advance ethical decisions and policymaking. After each report's release, the Bioethics Commission published educational materials to amplify its analysis and recommendations, making its work more accessible to diverse stakeholders (see Appendix II for a list of these materials).

The Bioethics Commission chose deliberation and education as the topic of its capstone report to underscore the importance it places on these two tools. To develop the recommendations contained in this report, the Bioethics Commission conducted four public meetings, heard from more than 20 experts, received numerous thoughtful public comments, and drew from its own experience on the topic of deliberation and education in bioethics. The report offers eight recommendations to advance the use of both tools as they intersect with bioethics.

CHAPTER 2
Democratic Deliberation in Bioethics

[D]eliberating with other human beings is the morally only
and best way we have in order to find good solutions to the
challenges for our societies and our global community.[17]

—Christianne Woopen, Chair, German Ethics Council, 2012–present

Democratic deliberation is a method of decision making in which participants discuss and debate a question of common concern, justifying their arguments with reasons and treating one another with mutual respect, with the goal of reaching an actionable decision for policy or law, open to future challenge or revision.[18] The process of democratic deliberation is especially useful for the types of ethical questions we face in bioethics, in which solutions have complex empirical as well as moral bases and about which reasonable people disagree. Bioethics advisory bodies can play a key role in leading these deliberations on the local, state, national, and international levels.

Although democratic deliberation can—and should—occur at all levels of decision making across a wide range of matters of common concern, we focus in this report on democratic deliberation in the areas of health, science, and technology policy for two reasons. First, these areas are the focus of bioethics and represent the topics on which the Bioethics Commission is best able to make a contribution in leading and supporting democratic deliberation. Second, topics in these areas are particularly well-suited to the process of democratic deliberation. They often are unsettled, become contentious, have public impact, and need public guidance to chart a path forward.

Effective democratic deliberation calls for inclusive and respectful debate and depends on collaborative decision making. Stakeholders with a range of perspectives are encouraged to present their views, seek common ground whenever possible, and maintain mutual respect even when irreconcilable differences among viewpoints remain.[19] *Deliberation* is distinct from the broader notion of *discussion*. A major goal of discussion is to develop an understanding of a topic. Deliberation includes understanding and adds the goal of arriving at a shared policy or course of action in response to a particular question of the form, "What should we do about this?"[20] The notion of collaborative decision making and inclusion of a range of perspectives is especially important when deliberating about bioethics. Bioethics is inherently interdisciplinary and involves questions of broad public concern that can be technical and complicated, both scientifically and ethically. Effective deliberation about these topics requires careful presentation and analysis of information as well as inclusion of all relevant viewpoints and stakeholders, from scientists and health care providers who are experts in the technology or policy being deliberated, to members of the public who will be affected by a decision, to professionals across a diversity of fields who can understand the implications of a policy for the law, industry, government, and beyond.

Democratic deliberation has played a vital role for bioethics bodies both inside and outside the United States as they formulate public policy on morally complex bioethical questions. For example, a national-level deliberation in the United Kingdom considered the implications of a new scientific technology that could prevent certain devastating diseases caused by failing mitochondria, the engine of cells, that can be passed on to children by the mitochondria in the mother's egg cell.[21] An estimated 1 in 5,000 individuals suffer from mitochondrial disease, which can cause damage to the brain, heart, liver, and kidneys.[22] The method honed in 2010 involves transferring the nucleus of the mother's egg cell into a donor egg that has healthy mitochondria. In 2012, the United Kingdom's

> "[B]ioethics is simply too important to be left to the bioethicists, but should offer opportunities for the general public to engage on a broad array of pertinent issues and to articulate their beliefs, secular or religious, and their concerns, be they related to technology or social injustices."
>
> Levin, D., Associate Professor, Department of Political Science, University of Utah. (2014). Deliberation and Bioethics Education: Overview. Presentation to the Bioethics Commission, November 6. Retrieved March 22, 2016 from http://bioethics.gov/node/4321.

Human Fertilisation and Embryology Authority (HFEA)—an independent regulatory agency for research and treatment involving embryos, sperm, and eggs—was asked by the government to assess public views on mitochondrial donation.[23] Through this project, HFEA hoped to "stimulate a rich and varied public debate, to help [it] make an informed decision" about regulations for this promising new intervention.[24] HFEA partnered with Sciencewise, a U.K. publicly funded national center for public dialogue in science and technology policy, to design a 13-month public dialogue process by using deliberative workshops, open consultation meetings, a representative survey, patient focus groups, and an open consultation questionnaire.[25]

At the conclusion of this process, HFEA reported that public deliberations had demonstrated that "general support [existed and]…that ethical concerns are outweighed by the arguments in favour of mitochondria replacement."[26] Drawing on HFEA's work, results of the public dialogue process, and input from the Nuffield Council on Bioethics, legislators developed the necessary infrastructure to regulate mitochondrial donation. Regulations were approved by U.K.'s Parliament in 2015.[27]

The process of democratic deliberation can serve both instrumental and expressive purposes: through deliberation, decision makers can ensure that decisions are based on relevant facts that have been subjected to reasoned judgment, serving the instrumental purpose of reaching better policy outcomes. A mutually respectful process also serves the expressive purpose of including and respecting affected stakeholders in the decision-making process, ensuring that decisions and policies are justifiable to those who will be affected by them.[28]

Democratic deliberation is not foolproof—limitations and challenges exist with every method of decision making. For example, reaching consensus can be difficult and the process misused to mask differences rather than understanding them. However, in general and compared with the status quo in our U.S. political system, deliberation has many advantages. It provides a morally and practically defensible way for addressing hyperpartisan gridlock. It also promotes mutual respect rather than fueling the sharp polarization and heightened differences that make consensus and legitimate outcomes nearly impossible in our current context.

A central tenet of democratic deliberation is reason-giving. Participants in deliberation are expected to offer reasons for their arguments and views and to incorporate the facts offered by opposing views into their reasoning.[29] This reciprocal reasoning has four fundamental features: accessibility, moral quality, respect, and revisability.[30] A deliberative exercise used in health care policymaking illustrates these four features. "Choosing Healthplans All Together" (CHAT), developed by Susan Goold, Marion Danis, and colleagues, uses a deliberative approach to engage participants in making complex decisions about which benefits to include in a health insurance package (Figure 2). During the exercise, participants move from making decisions individually, as if choosing coverage for themselves or their families, to choosing on behalf of a small community, to deciding on behalf of all members of a defined population (e.g., a state).[31] The results of CHAT exercises have guided decisions about health care prioritization, including capturing the health care coverage preferences of such underrepresented groups as low-income, uninsured individuals and older Medicare enrollees; streamlining employer-offered insurance; and developing innovative, collaborative insurance pools.[32]

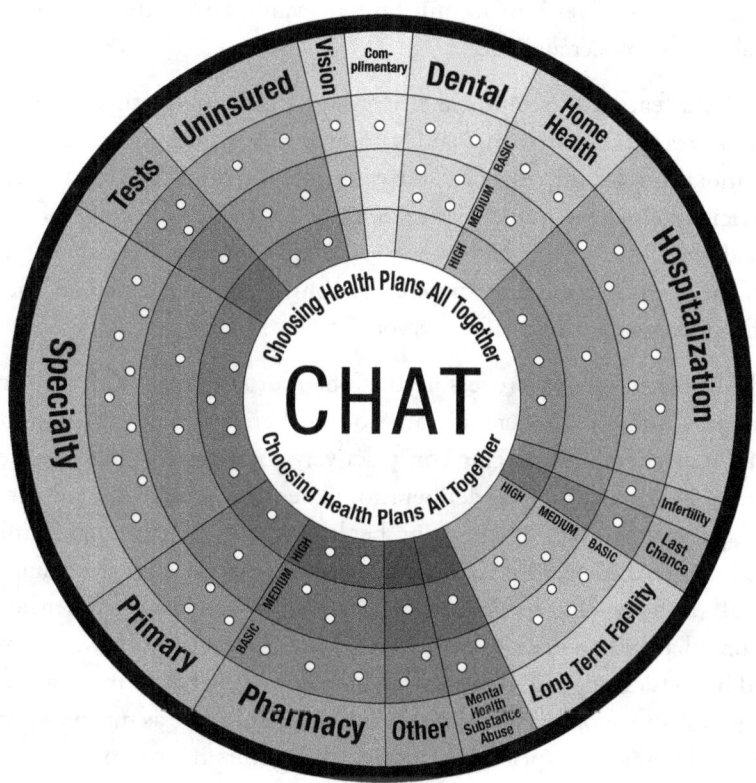

FIGURE 2: CHAT WHEEL

"Choosing Healthplans All Together" (CHAT) is a structured small-group deliberative exercise in which participants use the board pictured here to make decisions about health coverage for themselves and for the public. Source: Danis, M., Head, Section on Ethics and Health Policy, Department of Bioethics, National Institutes of Health (NIH) Clinical Center. (2015). Facilitating Public Dialogue about Bioethics. Presentation to the Bioethics Commission, September 2. Retrieved March 23, 2016, from http://bioethics.gov/node/5265.

The first feature of reciprocal reasoning is that the reasons given are *accessible* to everyone, which rules out, for example, reasons that appeal only to members of the population who hold certain beliefs (e.g., those with a particular religious belief) or scientific findings expressed in terms that are not intelligible to attentive laypersons. By asking individuals to make health coverage decisions on behalf of entire communities or populations, the CHAT exercise forces participants to incorporate others' perspectives. At the beginning of the exercise, when they are choosing health plans only for themselves, they can make decisions solely on the basis of their own values, but after they have to take other perspectives into account, the relevant reasons they give must be accessible to a broader audience.

The second feature of reciprocal reasoning is that the justifications given are *moral* reasons, in that they apply to everyone who is situated similarly in all morally relevant respects. For example, during the CHAT exercise, if participants believe that they are morally entitled to coverage of certain medical services, they should then extrapolate that moral reasoning to the rest of the community and the population, building that entitlement into the benefits package they design for everyone.

Third, the reason-giving process needs to be mutually *respectful*, an element that requires more than mere tolerance or indifference to others' viewpoints. Mutual respect entails engaging constructively with those who hold differing positions. Again, in CHAT deliberations, because participants must take on others' perspectives by choosing health plans for entire communities, individuals gain respect for their fellow participants because the results will affect all of them. One element of respect involves avoiding winner-take-all solutions that preference the majority opinion over others. Minority views should be considered, and solutions should be found that both impinge as little as possible on the dominant point of view and that satisfy as much as possible the minority goals. Respecting minority viewpoints instead of discounting them demonstrates respect for all participants in a deliberative process.

Finally, the conclusions reached need be *revisable* over time: a mechanism must be in place to revisit decisions in light of new information or conditions. The science or technology in question might advance, the context might change, or our understanding of the values at stake might shift with time.

Revisability allows decision makers to respond to these changes and ensures that all aspects of a decision, including norms, values, and theoretical commitments, are open to future challenge and subsequent revision or rejection if they no longer withstand scrutiny.[33] Policymakers who have used CHAT have noted that they must continue to revisit the deliberations and perhaps conduct new exercises to determine if the social climate has changed, especially when new information comes to light (e.g., new approved medical procedures or a shift in cultural norms).

> "Everywhere around the world...we found [that] people are smart if you create the conditions for collective deliberation.... The public is not stupid. It's just, normally, they're not paying attention. So if you can give them a reason [to] think their voice matters, they do very well."
>
> Fishkin, J.S., Janet M. Peck Professor of International Communication, Director, Center for Deliberative Democracy, Stanford University. (2015). Connecting Democratic Deliberation Theory to Practice. Presentation to the Bioethics Commission, May 27. Retrieved March 23, 2016 from http://bioethics.gov/node/4944.

These four features of reciprocal reasoning are essential in deliberations about bioethics. Bioethical concerns, which often involve matters of life and death, can evoke strong personal responses, and those participating in deliberations might have strong feelings about and be deeply invested in their views. These concerns are often also profoundly communal and collective, implicating moral questions, about what we owe each other in a just society, or what it means to be human. In the face of such questions, which are at once deeply personal and social, reciprocal reasoning requires that participants enter the deliberative process willing to respect those with different views and willing to give accessible reasons for their arguments rather than relying on personal beliefs or individual circumstances. Revisability is also important in bioethics deliberation, because bioethics often involves emerging technologies that, along with our understanding of them, are likely to evolve rapidly.

> "[D]eliberation does something. People change their minds after they deliberate."
>
> De Vries, R., Professor of Learning Health Sciences; Co-Director, Center for Bioethics and Social Sciences in Medicine; Professor of Sociology; Professor of Obstetrics and Gynecology, University of Michigan. (2015). Fostering and Measuring Success in Ethics and Deliberation. Presentation to the Bioethics Commission, September 2. Retrieved March 23, 2016 from http://bioethics.gov/node/5268.

The field of bioethics is often called upon to resolve seemingly intractable ethical conflicts and challenges.[34] Distributing scarce health resources, determining which patient should receive an organ available for transplant, or determining when restricting individuals' liberty for the community's safety and wellbeing is justifiable are central questions in bioethics that cannot be resolved except through a process in which multiple perspectives are shared and considered. These debates occur at all governmental levels in addition to communities, hospitals, institutional review boards, and professional societies. Deliberation is an essential process for finding points of agreement and moving forward on these morally complex concerns in all of these contexts.

In a deliberative democracy, the quality of deliberation legitimates the resulting consensus.[35] In contrast with outcomes determined by the victor of a battle of wills and power, the outcomes of deliberation derive from and are legitimized by exercise of reason toward the common good.[36] Deliberation can also legitimate policy decisions for the public by incorporating citizen voices—the majority of which are often unheard amid the clamor of interest groups—into the policymaking process.[37]

"The process can also increase the likelihood the priorities will be acceptable to the public. We often hear the public feeling like someone else has imposed priorities on them, and the limits are simply somebody else's ill-conceived ideas. But to the extent that they are involved themselves in making these tough choices, they appreciate the decisions that are made."

Danis, M., Head, Section on Ethics and Health Policy, Department of Bioethics, National Institutes of Health (NIH) Clinical Center. (2015). Facilitating Public Dialogue about Bioethics. Presentation to the Bioethics Commission, September 2. Retrieved March 23, 2016 from http://bioethics.gov/node/5265.

Democratic deliberation encourages participants to view issues and questions from different perspectives.[38] As recognized by the moral philosopher John Stuart Mill, when an individual contributes to decisions that impact the public, he must, "weigh interests not his own; …be guided, in case of conflicting claims, by another rule than his private partialities; [and] apply, at every turn, principles and maxims which have for their reason of existence the common good…."[39] In the deliberative process, participants must look outside their own interests and consider matters of common concern from the perspective of the broader public interest—an aspect of deliberation that is featured prominently in the CHAT exercise, where participants must choose plans not simply for themselves, but for entire communities. Exercises like CHAT demonstrate how deliberative processes can help individuals consider others' positions when making collective decisions about matters of public concern;

such decisions will then be justifiable to and regarded as legitimate by those who are bound by them.

National bioethics bodies can help to facilitate the deliberative process.[40] When constituted in a balanced way, bioethics bodies are designed to be conducive to deliberation, with members from diverse backgrounds and disciplines engaging in reasoned give-and-take regarding matters of public concern.[41] Acting as a form of national conscience, bioethics commissions can provide a public forum for consideration of concerns that are too complex, divisive, or entwined in the hands of interest groups to be addressed meaningfully by the U.S. Congress or other decision-making bodies. In a *New York Times* article and in public comment to the Bioethics Commission, bioethics scholar Alexander Capron emphasized the Commission's role in introducing the ethical, social, and scientific implications of biomedical advancements to the public in an organized way so as to encourage broad democratic deliberation: "[W]e've come to rely on more diverse bodies, like the bioethics commissions that have advised successive presidents since 1979. The challenge for any commission is to move these issues out of federal meeting rooms and engage the general public in deliberating about them in town halls, churches, schools and living rooms across the nation. Experts can help clarify the issues but policymaking ought to arise from a more democratic process."[42]

Although deliberation cannot make otherwise incompatible views compatible, it can help clarify what is at stake, elucidate points of agreement, help decision makers assess the widest range of public-spirited positions, and determine how much weight should be afforded to the different expressed preferences.[43] The success of this process in dealing with inescapable disagreement demonstrates that on concerns of great public interest with weighty ethical dimensions democratic deliberation is an essential tool for building policy that reflects and responds to public views. Democratic deliberation contributes to constructive, ethical decision making by expanding and improving public discourse. Embedded within this process is mutual respect among citizens, which is a core value of our constitutional democracy.

At What Level Is Democratic Deliberation Useful?

Making decisions in a large and diverse democracy is complex. Important decisions need deliberative forums of various types and sizes. Democratic deliberation can occur in many ways and at different levels of decision making, including among international, national, state, and local bodies. It also happens in smaller community-level organizations (e.g., schools, churches, hospitals, and universities). These different deliberative levels and venues reflect the complexity of decision making in a democracy and can be understood as interacting parts of a larger deliberative system that also accommodates other forms of decision making.[44]

"[T]he kinds of public deliberation about bioethics and regarding bioethics within the government is not and cannot and should not be restricted to groups with bioethics in their name or bioethics in their mandates; that these kinds of questions are present throughout the government's day-to-day work in health and medicine and not just in the obvious issues around genetics and pandemic preparedness and things like that, but how the FDA [Food and Drug Administration] weighs the risks and benefits of individual pharmaceuticals, how we debate the quality of evidence regarding preventative strategies, how we think about prioritizing vaccines as part of the recommended vaccination schedule."

Schwartz, J., Harold T. Shapiro Fellow in Bioethics, University Center for Human Values, Princeton University. (2015). Roundtable Discussion with the Bioethics Commission, May 27. Retrieved March 24, 2016 from http://bioethics.gov/node/4946.

The Bioethics Commission is a federal advisory committee and, as such, has deliberative features built into its structure. The Federal Advisory Committee Act—the act that governs all federal advisory committees—requires that committee meetings be open to the public with sufficient prior public notice; that those who are interested be permitted to attend, appear, or file comments with a committee; and that documents made available to or prepared for and by a committee be publically accessible.[45] Given its charge and its defined function under the act, the Bioethics Commission has deliberated publicly about many pressing questions of public concern. In the case of pediatric medical countermeasures, described in the following section, the deliberative function of the Bioethics Commission facilitated uptake of one of its key recommendations by other agencies across the federal government.

Deliberation also can occur on a global scale. World Wide Views, an organization supported by the Danish Board of Technology, has developed a method for hosting citizen deliberations on a global scale around a particular topic.[46] For example, the most recent global deliberation gathered 10,000 individuals at 97 sites across 76 countries to discuss climate and energy.[47] At each site, organizers recruited 100 participants of representative diversity, provided them with educational preparatory materials, presented key policy questions for moderated groups of five to eight participants across five sessions, and asked those participants to vote on the questions at the end of each session.[48] Key findings from the deliberations were connected to policymaking through presentations in New York City at the United Nations and in Paris at events surrounding the 2015 United Nations Climate Change Conference.[49] Previous World Wide Views deliberations have included global climate change and biodiversity. These global events demonstrate that individuals from diverse nations can participate in meaningful deliberations involving policy concerns at the nexus of science and ethics. Such a model can be extended to other pressing bioethics topics.

Highly controversial questions also have been deliberated at the state level. The ethical questions of if and when life-sustaining treatments for critically ill patients should be removed and who should make such decisions have challenged bioethicists, health care workers, and family members for decades. The New York State Task Force on Life and the Law dealt with this topic and published multiple reports tackling it from different angles, including a report about do-not-resuscitate orders, one about physician-assisted dying, and another about appointing surrogates for making decisions about end-of-life sustaining treatment when the patient is unable to communicate.[50]

The Task Force is an example of a body designed to deliberate on the ethical dimensions of law and policy at the state level. It was established by Governor Mario Cuomo in 1985 and is a standing body consisting of 23 appointed experts who volunteer their time to assist the state in developing public policy regarding the interface of medicine, law, and ethics. The Task Force comprises leaders in religion, philosophy, law, medicine, nursing, and bioethics and is chaired by New York State's Commissioner of Health.[51] It has produced influential reports on cutting-edge bioethics topics, including surrogate consent for human subjects research, assisted reproductive technologies, organ transplantation, dietary supplements, genetic testing, and allocation of ventilators during an influenza pandemic.[52] Ten of the Task Force's recommendations have been adopted as legislation or regulation in New York, and they have substantially affected health care delivery in the state. Additionally, other states, including Georgia, Illinois, Massachusetts, and Vermont, have embraced the Task Force's recommendations as models for their own legislation.[53]

At the institutional level, hospital ethics committees bring together a range of perspectives and voices from within the institution to deliberate policies relevant to its functioning. These committees can serve both educational and advisory purposes. Hospital ethics committees typically include physicians, nurses, and other health care professionals who have an interest in ethics.[54] The committees also might include patient representatives or community members who are not hospital staff.[55] A central function of hospital ethics committees is to assist in resolving complex ethical problems that arise during care and treatment of individual patients in the institution. Although individual cases are decided privately, not deliberated publicly, recommendations of ethics committees also are used to guide institutional policies that have complex ethical dimensions (e.g., patients' rights, end-of-life decisions, and staff and family conflicts).[56]

How Does Democratic Deliberation Work?

As a public advisory body, the Bioethics Commission has used deliberative processes to formulate recommendations regarding some of the country's most challenging bioethical dilemmas. Although context, topic, timeline, resources, and other variables can affect how democratic deliberation is conducted, the deliberative process should have certain general features that can be adapted to suit the needs and goals of a particular group. In the case of the Bioethics Commission, the features are illustrated by the steps followed in our deliberation on pediatric countermeasure research. In 2013, the Bioethics Commission released its report on research with children to study medical countermeasures for use in the event of a bioterrorist attack: *Safeguarding Children: Pediatric Medical Countermeasure Research* (*Safeguarding Children*).[57]

The process of democratic deliberation was essential to arriving at recommendations that all members could support and that could have a critically important practical impact. After more than a year of intense deliberation that included four public meetings and input from diverse experts and stakeholders, the Bioethics Commission recommended that testing of medical countermeasures be conducted by using progressive age de-escalation (see following Text Box). The Biomedical Advanced Research and Development Authority and the Centers for Disease Control and Prevention subsequently conducted a study of anthrax vaccine that provided the basis for using informed age de-escalation with pediatric research participants.[58] The uptake of this recommendation demonstrates that public deliberation can be an effective process for finding a reasoned way forward on some of the most morally controversial and difficult science policy questions that our society faces. This process followed the steps for deliberation outlined in this section. Examples of real deliberation from those meetings are displayed in Figure 3. The following steps serve as a guide for those planning a deliberative activity as they make choices about the design of the process.

PROGRESSIVE AGE DE-ESCALATION

In its report *Safeguarding Children: Pediatric Medical Countermeasure Research*, the Bioethics Commission recommended that pre-event pediatric medical countermeasure research proceed through progressive age de-escalation whenever possible. By assessing and evaluating risks from a group of young adults, age de-escalation can be used to guide the research design and the estimate of risk level for a group of older children; those results can be used to characterize the research risks for the next younger age group, and so forth. This recommendation represents a compromise between those who believe that being prepared for an emergency is of the utmost importance, even if research poses more than minimal risk, and those who believe that it is never acceptable to expose children to more than minimal risk without the prospect of direct benefit.

Presidential Commission for the Study of Bioethical Issues (PCSBI). (2013, March). *Safeguarding Children: Pediatric Medical Countermeasure Research*. Washington, DC: PCSBI.

Begin with an Open Question and Consider Distinct Points of View

Democratic deliberation is best suited for questions or complex topics with no clear consensus about a way forward. One bioethics topic particularly well-suited for democratic deliberation is surrogate consent for participation in research. This topic has been debated for decades and, although progress has been made toward resolving the questions of if and how surrogate consent might be provided for participation in research, questions remain. As the Bioethics Commission recognized in its report, *Gray Matters: Topics at the Intersection of Neuroscience, Ethics, and Society*, legal guidance on this topic is inadequate and varies considerably by state.[59] Research indicates that when members of the public are given the opportunity to engage in a deliberative discussion about this topic, considerable progress can be made toward practical solutions.[60] The Bioethics Commission modeled democratic deliberation on this topic at the federal policy level and succeeded in influencing federal policy in the form of a proposed change to the interpretation of human subjects protection regulations.[61] Because state and local laws and policies are also involved, continued deliberation at other levels is necessary—in fact, the New York State Task Force, described in the previous section, also confronted this question and succeeded in changing relevant state policies. The problem of consent capacity demonstrates that a topic might be well-suited for deliberation at one level, but the relevant questions and goals on the same topic might vary when deliberated at another level.

Similar to the question of surrogate consent for research, topics for deliberation should allow for discussions that are not purely theoretical; rather, the topics in question should have practical implications—deliberations should involve questions about how we can move forward and what should be done.[62] As Figure 3 illustrates, the question of medical countermeasure research, and specifically if pediatric research on the anthrax vaccine should proceed, was a complex and challenging topic that required a practical answer and a path forward.

FIGURE 3

STEPS FOR DELIBERATION

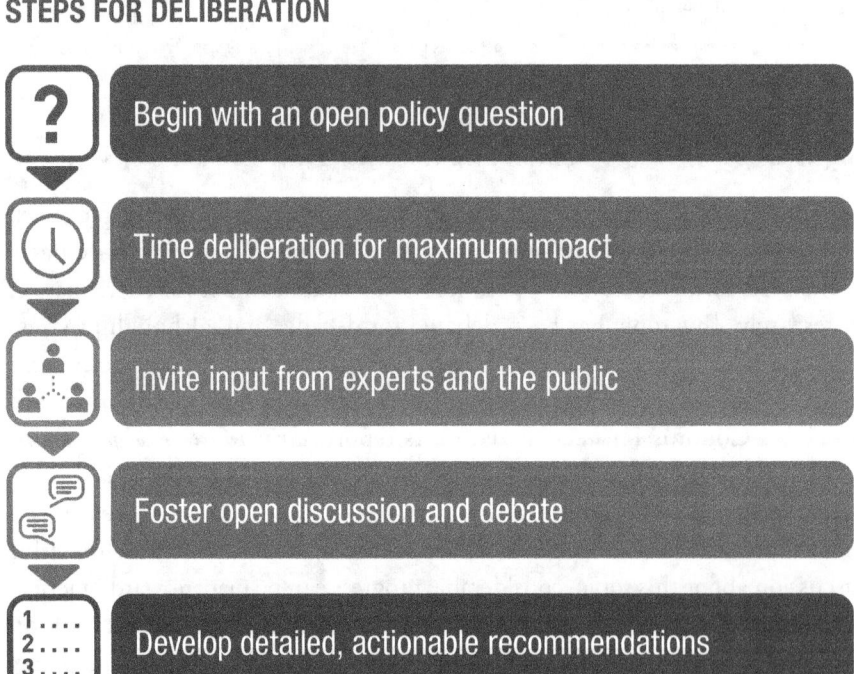

STEPS FOR DELIBERATION – EXAMPLE IN ACTION
Safeguarding Children: Pediatric Medical Countermeasure Research

 National Biodefense Science Board, October 2011 · Before an anthrax attack occurs, should pediatric research testing the safety and degree of immune response to an anthrax vaccine go forward? "The issue should be referred to an appropriate review board to formally address the ethical considerations. This board should include ethicists and public representation."

 Letter from Kathleen Sebelius, Secretary of Health and Human Services, to the Bioethics Commission, January 2012 · "Given the complexity and sensitivity of this issue, I ask that the Commission consult with a range of experts within and outside the United States Government, to include the medical and scientific communities in addition to non-profit organizations and other public constituencies. I ask that the Commission provide me with a report of its findings, as well as any recommendations and suggestions the Commission deems appropriate. I would welcome the opportunity to further discuss a timeframe for this project that is mutually agreeable, taking into consideration both the urgency and complexity of the issue."

 Commission Meeting, May 2012 · *Dr. Gutmann, Chair:* Is there a vaccine, anthrax vaccine for adults, and does that allow us to extrapolate that there could be a safe one developed that could be tested at minimal risk for children? In other words, that's a big question but I think we need some baseline here as to what the factual records suggests about one of the questions we're very specifically being asked to answer.

Dr. Robert Nelson, Senior Pediatric Ethicist/Lead Medical Officer, Office of Pediatric Therapeutics, Office of the Commissioner, Food and Drug Administration: The anthrax vaccine is approved for adults for prevention. I mean, it's disbursed in the military and given under that indication…In other words, in the case of an event, you would then deliver it…There's no data in pediatrics at all.

Commission Meeting, November 2012 · *Bruce Lockwood, Vice President, USA Council of International Association of Emergency Managers:* Absent the security of prepositioned antibiotics in-home, pre-event vaccines, and increased awareness about the need to simultaneously protect first responders and their households, there is a distinct possibility for degraded emergency services. The potential for this cascading effect keeps me awake at night. It also underscores the necessity for the development of a pathway for licensing vaccines, including AVA for children.

Commission Meeting, November 2012 · *Dr. Gutmann, Chair:* We don't want to begin with a statement up front that basically decides issues, as opposed to opening our minds and any groups' minds to thinking about all of the steps that have to go through.

Dr. Arras, Member: This research will give us a smidgeon of the evidence. It is not going to tell us whether this particular vaccine is safe or effective…it is going to give us just one small step in that direction, which a lot of our panelists said, well, you know, it is better than nothing and you've got to start somewhere.

Dr. Kucherlapati, Member: The goal for society as a whole is to try to keep all of the population, including the children, to be as healthy as possible…There is no human enterprise that is completely devoid of risk. And so one has to be willing to accept some level of risk and I don't know what that level of risk is.

 Safeguarding Children Report, March 2013 · The Bioethics Commission concluded that higher risk is unacceptable in pre-event research as such research does not directly benefit the child participants and the likelihood that the results of such research would benefit other children is unknown or unknowable…. Minimal risk pediatric research should employ progressive age de-escalation whenever possible, from the oldest group of children to the youngest. p. 20, p. 4

Debates that involve deep disagreement and seemingly incompatible moral values, but that also have broad public impact and require concrete action, are particularly suitable for democratic deliberation in which the emphasis is on providing mutually acceptable justifications for the policy to those who will be bound by it.[63] The Community Ethics Committee in Boston, a group of citizens who provide feedback to Harvard teaching hospitals on policies with ethical dimensions, is an example of how diverse members of the community can deliberate to propose answers to emotionally charged and value-laden ethical questions. One such topic addressed by the Community Ethics Committee was whether pediatric patients with neurodevelopmental disabilities should be treated differently than other patients when listing them for organ transplantation.[64] The Committee's process included hearing from individuals and family members affected by the discussion topic, followed by deliberation regarding responses to the challenging ethical question.[65] Interdisciplinary deliberation similar to that of the Community Ethics Committee can produce nuanced responses to problems, drawing from relevant expertise across many perspectives.[66]

Democratic deliberation is especially effective for decisions and policies related to emerging technologies. Advances in science, medicine, and technology offer tremendous promise and potential benefits to individuals and society and also pose known and unknown risks, especially when their consequences are not yet well-understood. Because of their novelty, emerging technologies present uncertainty, which can make calculating how to promote innovation while also minimizing harm difficult. Thus, careful and iterative review is necessary. Deliberation among the scientific community, policymakers, and the public fosters open debate, helps educate stakeholders and the public, and ensures that a broad constituency is represented in the outcome. It can be a helpful approach to monitoring and facilitating use of emerging technologies.[67] Typically, democratic deliberation about ethical controversies gives voice to the public's views about content and application of ethical norms and facilitates the public's standing in health and technology policy.

"The first and, in many ways, I think the most important [reason for public engagement], is to hear the often unheard voices, by which I mean that often silent majority of people beyond the organized and vociferous stakeholder groups."

Jackson, R., Executive Chair, Sciencewise. (2015). Facilitating Public Dialogue about Bioethics. Presentation to the Bioethics Commission September 2. Retrieved March 25, 2016 from http://bioethics.gov/node/5265.

Time the Deliberation for Maximum Impact

Deliberation optimally is conducted when a topic is ripe for discussion—meaning relevant facts are established—and ready for potential policy change—meaning an opportunity exists to make a decision and change a policy or law in response to the deliberation. Enough time to deliberate should be available before a decision becomes absolutely necessary. When the Bioethics Commission deliberated about pediatric medical countermeasures in 2012, the fundamental question was whether research with children to determine safety and effectiveness of the anthrax vaccine for individuals aged less than 18 years should be conducted before a potential bioterrorist attack occurs. The anthrax vaccine is currently approved for use in adults only.[68] These deliberations were conducted with time to make a reasoned and ethical decision and to have a new policy in place before an attack occurs (Figure 3).

Because pre-decisional timing is impossible in the midst of an emergency, ensuring that public officials anticipate and are vigilant about ethical challenges that might arise during an emergency is all the more important. Engaging in deliberative discussions in advance will aid decision making when an emergency does arise. In its report *Ethics and Ebola: Public Health Planning and Response* (*Ethics and Ebola*), the Bioethics Commission considered some of these challenges as they arose during the 2014–2016 Ebola epidemic in western Africa. It recognized that democratic deliberation is key to preparedness for future public health emergencies, given that the success of public health policies depends, in large part, on their perceived legitimacy to individuals and communities most affected by them. Decisions made both before and during public health emergencies, particularly related to measures that might restrict individuals' liberties, should be deliberated democratically to ensure that they are viewed as legitimate, supported by reasons that include best-available scientific and public health evidence, and can be revisited in light of rapidly changing information.[69] To the extent possible, deliberation should be conducted in advance of an emergency because it might be impossible while the emergency is ongoing.

Experiences on the ground in western Africa during the Ebola epidemic demonstrate that, even in the midst of a devastating public health crisis, committing time and resources to public deliberation is both possible and productive. In Liberia, UNICEF (United Nations) rapid-response teams engaged with communities in some of the most devastated areas through house-to-house visits, town hall meetings, and focus group discussions about urgent concerns, including prevention measures, reporting and isolation of ill family members, burial practices, and stigma.[70] In Guinea, the Centers for Disease Control and Prevention (U.S.) worked with community members to host seven town hall meetings with more than 1,000 participants, each of which lasted until every participant's concern and question had been addressed.[71] These efforts highlight the importance of creating opportunities for communities to deliberate together on the most urgent matters of common concern, even in the midst of an emergency.

Invite Input from Experts and the Public

Establishing the scientific and other empirical evidence about a topic is an essential step in the democratic deliberation process. Sometimes, new information will emerge during deliberations, or existing information will change. Figure 3 illustrates Commission members learning new information from experts in real time around the deliberation table. The task of gathering facts is best understood not as a step that is performed once at the outset of the deliberation, but rather as an iterative process where relevant information aids the deliberation as new facts emerge. Moreover, those leading or participating in the deliberation might disagree about the facts of a given topic. Ensuring all purported facts are checked through an established and reliable mechanism is an essential step to take both before and during deliberation. Providing established facts in the form of accessible background materials available to all participants is important before starting deliberation, but it is equally important during deliberation as well.[72]

In its own work, the Bioethics Commission has dealt first hand with the challenge of establishing the facts around a question while engaging in its deliberation. When conducting its deliberations on the applications of neuroscience to the legal system, the Bioethics Commission aspired to use substantiated facts to avoid using exaggerated or unverified scientific claims. The Bioethics Commission noted in its report on neuroscience that, especially in the courtroom where life and liberty are at stake, the expert invocation of unsubstantiated facts or unverified scientific conclusions is ethically indefensible. Sometimes, review of the literature revealed two or three published articles describing neuroscience findings linking, for example, a particular brain region with violent or impulsive behavior. Rather than assuming that this kind of evidence was ready for use as evidence in a criminal trial, the Bioethics Commission endeavored to investigate whether findings were validated, replicated, or challenged by other studies. Using reliable and validated scientific facts allowed the Bioethics Commission to make practical and reasoned recommendations regarding use of neuroscience in the courtroom, including a recommendation to avoid overstatement and unfounded conclusions.[73]

When deliberating while information is rapidly changing, establishing facts as much as possible at the outset is crucial; however, willingness to adapt to changing circumstances and reestablish agreed-upon facts, if they change, is also essential. As described previously, in *Ethics and Ebola* the Bioethics Commission discussed the importance of democratic deliberation before and during a public health emergency, acknowledging the challenges of deliberating while information is rapidly changing.[74] Even outside of the emergency context, facts and circumstances sometimes change during the course of or after a deliberation. Designed to deal with the dual complexities of social change and imperfect knowledge, deliberative bodies can always welcome improved and updated information to better guide their ongoing deliberations.

For a structured deliberative activity, background materials should be prepared by objective parties or by experts holding various views on a contested topic. The materials also might include a reasoned argument on different sides of a question, to model for participants how to use established facts and ethics principles to form opinions with fully formed justifications. However, deciding what to include in these materials—that is, deciding what the established facts are—is not always straightforward. Reaching agreement between experts on what constitutes balanced and accurate information might be difficult, particularly when the topic is new or controversial or when those preparing the materials are invested in particular views.[75] The Bioethics Commission strived to achieve a balanced and objective gathering of evidence by hearing from a diverse set of experts during its public meetings. These experts reflected the interdisciplinary nature of the relevant topics. Often the panelists disagreed with one another, and listening to the reasons they gave for their positions helped Commission members form or modify their own views.

> "[D]eliberation needs facts, but it doesn't end with facts. The issues are too important to be left for scientific experts."
>
> Thompson, D., Alfred North Whitehead Professor of Political Philosophy, Faculty of Arts and Sciences; Professor of Public Policy, John F. Kennedy School of Government, Harvard University (Emeritus). (2015). Facilitating Public Dialogue about Bioethics. Presentation to the Bioethics Commission, September 2. Retrieved March 25, 2016 from http://bioethics.gov/node/5265.

Multiple factors should be considered when deciding whom and how many individuals to include as participants in a deliberative process. For national deliberative polls, which do not usually involve deliberative decision making but often inform decision makers, the aim is for the participants to reflect the nation's population.[76] This might mean selecting as many as 500 individuals, either randomly or through stratified random sampling to ensure that those selected reflect the nation's diversity.[77] For deliberative processes that fulfill the decision-making function of deliberation, groups made up of one or two dozen participants can strike a good balance between including differing perspectives while maximizing efficiency and minimizing cost.[78]

Foster Open Discussion and Debate

Mutual respect and reason-giving are two principal values of democratic deliberation. Mutual respect serves both instrumental and ethical functions. It enables more effective deliberation because it enhances communication and leads to more compromise and productive solutions. It also reflects the value of community members with diverse perspectives participating together in the governance of a pluralistic society.[79]

Similarly, reason-giving has both instrumental and ethical functions. Instrumentally, it helps those engaged in deliberation come to a decision based on reasoned arguments that can be justified to and regarded as legitimate by those who will be bound by it. Ethically, it reflects the value of community members as participants in their democracy. Rather than being treated merely as "objects of legislation," it ensures that they engage with the

> "[A]verage people whose daily lives don't get them involved in decision making like is happening here, they are just doing their jobs, raising their families, living their lives—but they do have opinions, very strong opinions about the things they see in the paper or hear on the news. And so, if they are given information and opportunity, they can contribute to the wellbeing of all of us."
>
> Evans, F., Deliberative Poll Participant, What's Next California (2015). Facilitating Public Dialogue about Bioethics. Presentation to the Bioethics Commission, September 2. Retrieved March 25, 2016 from http://bioethics.gov/node/5265.

process and that legislators and other policymakers give and respond to reasons for laws and policies.[80]

Although the ideals of mutual respect and reason-giving can be challenging to maintain in the midst of a contentious deliberation, facilitators must create an environment that enables participants to practice these principles. Facilitators can be trained to nurture civility during deliberative proceedings.[81] Their prompts can encourage participants to express minority views, to provide reasons for their arguments, to consider the pros and cons of their own stances, and not to demand or expect that the group reach a consensus.[82]

"We stress mutual respect, however, because, even more than other ethical considerations, it is *intrinsically* a part of deliberation. To deliberate with another is to understand the other as a self-authoring source of reasons and claims. To fail to grant to another the moral status of authorship is, in effect, to remove oneself from the possibility of deliberative influence. By the same token, being open to being moved by the words of another is to respect the other as a source of reasons, claims, and perspectives."

Source: Mansbridge, J., et al. (2012). A Systemic Approach to Deliberative Democracy. In J. Parkinson and J. Mansbridge. (Eds.). *Deliberative Systems: Deliberative Democracy at the Large Scale* (pp. 1-26). New York, NY: Cambridge University Press, p. 11. [Original emphasis]

Develop Detailed, Actionable Recommendations

After a compromise, consensus, or agreement has emerged from the deliberation, the decisions made must be fed back into the decision- and policymaking processes, wherever possible. Deliberations can be linked to the policy process in different ways. For example, in the United Kingdom, the Sciencewise program was established with the explicit purpose of embedding public dialogue in the policymaking process.[83] Sciencewise provides advice and support directly to policymakers about how to conduct deliberative dialogue with the public on a topic, with the aim of ensuring that public dialogue is an integral part of policymaking. Findings from the public dialogue on mitochondria replacement were integrated back into the HFEA advice to the government, which in turn guided its decision to allow patients access to this new technology.[84] Notably, Sciencewise only engages with topics for deliberation about which policy decisions are not yet determined and can be influenced by public engagement. The legitimacy of the outcome of deliberations increases when stakeholders are involved in initiating and designing the activity.[85] In the United States, the Oregon Citizens' Initiative Review program selects citizens to deliberate and produce a written analysis about state ballot initiatives. The analysis is distributed in the official voters' pamphlet, linking the deliberation to the policy process.[86] Evaluation of the program revealed that a majority of Oregon voters were aware of the process, two-thirds of those reading its products regarded them as helpful for voting, and reading the analysis improved voter knowledge.[87]

Benefits of Democratic Deliberation

Democratic deliberation can help groups of citizens and decision makers reach consensus when other methods have failed. It also can help disparate groups arrive at decisions that are regarded as legitimate by all parties, even if not everyone agrees. It fosters mutual respect and understanding among individuals with diverse values and viewpoints. These benefits are illustrated by examining cases in which the *absence* of deliberation led to policies that likely *decreased* their public legitimacy. The well-publicized example of the development of the Oregon Health Plan—in which a vote by the state legislature was insufficient for the public to recognize a policy change as legitimate, but subsequent inclusion of the public in deliberation was well-received—merits an extended discussion, because it demonstrates the evolution of policy on a weighty topic as it is guided by public deliberation.

In 1989, Oregon converted its Medicaid program to the Oregon Health Plan, with the aim of expanding the program to all residents living in poverty. For more residents to receive this Medicaid coverage, the plan had to cover fewer medical procedures. The proposal created a ranking system of medical priorities—a list of all medical procedures ranked from most to least important. Medicaid would cover procedures to a certain point on the list determined by the Oregon legislature.[88]

Before the creation of this plan in July 1987, the Oregon state legislature voted to discontinue Medicaid funding for heart, liver, pancreas, and bone marrow transplants. These services were considered optional under federal Medicaid rules. The legislators justified the decision on the basis of the high costs and low success rates of those procedures, but they made the decision without input from the public or health care professionals.[89] Nationwide attention focused on this decision when Coby Howard, a 7-year-old male with leukemia, was denied funding for a bone-marrow transplant.[90] After he died, the Oregon legislature voted on a measure to appropriate $220,000 from the state's general fund to pay for transplants for the eight remaining individuals who had been denied funding under the new policy. The motion was defeated twice at the urging of then state senate president John Kitzhaber, an emergency department physician, who argued for development of an evidence-based policy for rationing health care.[91] Kitzhaber wanted to shift the debate over Medicaid funding to focus instead on what, rather than whom, the plan should cover.[92]

The proposed bill, the Oregon Basic Health Services Act, made provisions to expand state health care coverage to include all Oregonians living at or below 100% of the poverty level. The bill would create the Oregon Health Services Commission (HSC), an 11-member group comprising health care providers and consumers. The commission would compile "a list of health services ranked by priority, from the most important to the least important, representing the comparative benefits of each service to the population to be served."[93] HSC would create a new list every 2 years.[94] The Oregon legislature, provided with estimated costs of placing the funding level at each point on the list, would then determine how much of the list would be funded—where the cut-off point would be. It would remove the option of cutting program costs by changing eligibility restrictions or reimbursement rates. All services needed for establishing a diagnosis would be included, even if the treatment for the uncovered condition would cost less than the cut-off point.

Because the health services ranking list was the central component of the Oregon Health Plan, designers of the program believed that it should be developed using a method that would garner public confidence and trust. Hence, public participation in the ranking process was encouraged. The bill required that HSC have open meetings exclusively and sponsor forums for members of the public to contribute their views. A key lesson from public outcry over the earlier decisions to cut funding for transplantation of certain organs was that, for the policy to succeed, the public must be part of the decision-making process.[95]

HSC was required to hold public hearings to solicit input from "advocates for seniors; handicapped persons; mental health services consumers; low-income Oregonians; and providers of health care" and actively seek "consensus on the values to be used to guide health resource allocation decisions."[96] The public hearings were intended to provide an opportunity for groups with different views to express prioritization preferences. The community meetings where public involvement was solicited were intended as sessions for gathering information from the community about what values were important to the residents of the state.[97] A summary report detailed the 13 themes that members of the public thought should guide the ranking process, and in response to this report, HSC developed a new ranking process, based in large part on the public's input.[98] Even critics who might find the resulting coverage to be inadequate can acknowledge that a deliberative process better enables their criticisms to be brought to light.

Decisions that affect the deeply held values and welfare of the public, such as the allocation of scarce resources for competing health care priorities, cannot be left to policy- and lawmakers alone without input from the community and affected stakeholders. In the absence of democratic deliberation on policy matters of deep public interest, trust in the policymaking process is corroded. Including public consensus brought about through democratic deliberation helps create policies that are perceived as legitimate by the public, particularly when policy decisions have bioethical dimensions—affecting medical care, participation in research, and other questions of life and welfare. Thus, the Bioethics Commission makes three recommendations for increasing and improving use of democratic deliberation in bioethics, with particular focus on public policy with bioethical dimensions.

Recommendations

Earlier in this chapter, we described a recommendation in *Safeguarding Children* that the Bioethics Commission made after a year-long process of deliberation and that was subsequently implemented at the federal level. Such examples demonstrate the success of democratic deliberation in helping solve complex bioethical challenges. Developing legitimate policy solutions to these challenges requires listening to, considering, and incorporating diverse perspectives. Bioethical concerns are often polarizing and controversial, not unlike topics debated and discussed among politicians and on the national stage. Our role, as a nonpartisan bioethics commission, is to demonstrate respectful deliberation of controversial topics as an antidote to the polarized political climate, which is increasingly permeated by scapegoating, name-calling, and gridlock, while the urgency and depth of the problems faced by the public persist.

The following recommendations, if implemented, would enhance public dialogue and deliberation in circumstances in which complex ethical concerns are at stake, and would contribute to sound and legitimate public policy for health, science, and technology.

Recommendation 1: Guide Bioethics Policy Decisions with Democratic Deliberation

Stakeholders in the democratic process at all levels—including communities, policymakers, popular opinion leaders, and advisory bodies—should use a well-crafted form of democratic deliberation to inform and guide health, science, and technology policy decisions and their ethical dimensions. Policymakers, communities, and advisory bodies should use democratic deliberation to consider morally complex and controversial bioethical problems to promote mutual understanding and respect among participants as well as greater legitimacy for resulting policy.

Successful democratic deliberation fosters greater individual and mutual understanding of problems of common concern, broader public engagement with complex policy questions, and legitimacy of decision making. Both immediate and long-term benefits result from diverse stakeholders in our democracy participating in forums for decision making that reflect the core values of democratic deliberation.[99]

Democratic deliberations should occur at the different levels of decision making and involve the depth and breadth of stakeholders necessary to develop a way forward on difficult policy questions of broad societal import. Examples of deliberation occurring at different levels were described earlier in this chapter, including deliberations of this Bioethics Commission at the federal level, development of national regulations on mitochondrial donation in the United Kingdom, and other initiatives at the state, local, and community levels (e.g., the New York State Taskforce on Life and the Law), and in certain instances, by institutional ethics committees.

Well-designed deliberations, whether large or small, are structured to ensure that all participants are respected and engaged, that minority views and voices are heard, and that outcomes are the product of respectful and reasoned dialogue among participants with diverse backgrounds, expertise, and perspectives. The community consultation conducted by the Oregon Health

Services Commission in the late 1980s and early 1990s, described earlier in the chapter, is an example of a well-designed deliberation. The deliberative process was successful because it encouraged community members and policymakers to reflect on their values and arrive at a solution outside of their original predisposition in a way that left the public feeling respected and included in the process. Public deliberations like these are iterative processes, open to revision and self-correction.

From formal and structured deliberative polling activities to less formal community conversations, democratic deliberation is an effective element of decision making in many different contexts. An extensive body of research has been conducted during past decades to determine the methods for group communication and deliberation that are most effective and conducive to success. That research has resulted in a growing body of literature detailing effective methods and best practices for deliberation, some of which was summarized in the previous discussion. Those who organize and facilitate deliberative activities should review the process for democratic deliberation, including the sections presented previously on when and for what kinds of topics democratic deliberation should be conducted, how to conduct the deliberations, and how those deliberations can contribute to the policy process. Taking lessons from past successful—and unsuccessful—methods of deliberation will help organizers tailor their activities to the population who will participate and the topics under consideration.

Recommendation 2: Conduct Deliberative Activities in Ways Conducive to Mutual Respect and Reason-Giving Among Participants in Accordance with Best Practices

Organizers of deliberative activities should ensure that deliberation is accomplished in accordance with best practices established in the broad body of scholarly literature. At a minimum, effective deliberative processes require participants to give reasons for their arguments and to show respect for fellow participants. In addition, the set of concerns for deliberation should raise questions for which practical decisions need to be made, and the deliberations should be intended and designed to influence how those decisions are made.

Individuals and entities that organize deliberative processes, or would like to incorporate democratic deliberation into their decision-making processes, should review and incorporate existing literature on methods and best practices. Steps in the process were described previously and are included in Appendix I (Steps for Deliberation). Other considerations include how long to deliberate, how many individuals to include, whether to seek a random sample or ensure inclusion from members of certain groups, what preparatory materials to make available, and how to incorporate expert consultation and supply useful information for those engaged in deliberation. Regardless of variations in the deliberative process, at a minimum, it should require that participants give reasons for their views and show respect for one another. As a concrete demonstration of respect, decisions should aim, if possible, to enable minority practices to continue to flourish, provided these practices do not threaten the common good or unduly burden the majority's ability to implement the agreed-upon policy. Additional best practices will depend on the particular goals and context of the deliberative activity. For example, the 2014–2016 Ebola epidemic in western Africa raised ethically relevant policy questions regarding quarantine of returning health care workers and research conducted during a public health emergency. The Bioethics Commission recognized the need to respond to these pressing challenges swiftly and effectively through transparent, democratic, and public deliberation. The Bioethics Commission assembled a diverse group of experts and stakeholders, including representatives from affected communities, and adapted its deliberative process to meet an accelerated timeline.[100]

Democratic deliberation has been demonstrated to be an effective tool for facilitating public engagement and fostering an environment of mutual respect. But deliberation is not a one-size-fits-all process—it can involve substantially different variables and methods. Measures for comparing different deliberative methods and deliberative and non-deliberative processes of decision making should be developed to further support the goals of Recommendation 2. For example, many scholars agree that incorporating public opinion into bioethics scholarship and health policy development is important. Further research to determine the comparative value and success of deliberative activities in this context will help guide the process of soliciting public views and using them to best effect. One study, for example, compared the relative merits of opinion surveys versus deliberative processes for gauging the views of the public in decisions about how and whether to obtain surrogate consent for research participation.[101] The authors concluded that opinion surveys risk eliciting superficial and uninformed views that might be insufficient for guiding policymaking. Democratic deliberation, by contrast, ensures that participants are educated about the topic under discussion and its nuances and complexities, and by its very nature necessitates that participants give reasons for their views. More research on the effectiveness of deliberation will improve the empirical evidence for best practices in different contexts.

Recommendation 3: To Further the Practical Contribution of Deliberation in Bioethics, Conduct Additional Research on the Effectiveness of Deliberative Methods

Scholars of democratic deliberation, along with individuals and organizations using democratic deliberation for decision making, should continue to assess the effectiveness of particular deliberative methods as tools to address complex bioethical challenges. These studies should evaluate the processes and outcomes of different kinds of deliberation and establish measurements of success.

During the past decade, scholars have begun to develop and refine measures for evaluating the effectiveness of deliberative activities.[102] In evaluating these activities, they have been attentive to both processes and outcomes, but more work remains. Specifically, formative and process evaluations should include questions about how to conduct democratic deliberation to maximize mutual respect, optimize engagement, and elicit less commonly held perspectives to create an inclusive discussion of policy proposals. Public health policies are a particularly important area for public deliberation because they require cooperation among substantial portions of the population. A deliberative approach that engages affected communities and uses deliberative processes to reach policy solutions that are both ethically and scientifically sound leads to public health policies with greater legitimacy for those most affected by them.

Evaluation of the outcomes of public deliberation should include an understanding about how to design deliberative activities to produce the desired goals. Goals include a more informed voting public, a potential policy change, and a greater public sense of inclusion in law and policy decisions. An inclusive and broadly shared framework for evaluating both processes and outcomes of deliberation would be a valuable tool to encourage policymakers and other leaders to use democratic deliberation as an integral part of the decision-making process. Empirical evidence regarding what works and what does not—with a focus on how to change what does not—is essential to implementing sound strategies to improve public policy.[103]

* * *

Deliberation is especially necessary in our current and increasingly polarized political climate. As science and technology rapidly advance, often what we technically *can* do becomes clear before we have assessed what we ethically *should* do. In these areas, deeply held personal values are at play, life and death can be at stake, and the addition of perspectives from diverse stakeholders and public citizens can enrich and add legitimacy to policy decisions. Well-reasoned and effective deliberation about bioethics is not possible without participants who are educated about the relevant science and technology and who are clear about the values they bring to the discussion. Ethics education is necessary for effective democratic deliberation about bioethics—a topic addressed in the next chapter of this report.

CHAPTER 3
Bioethics Education

> *We must remember that intelligence is not enough.*
> *Intelligence plus character—that is the goal of true education.*
> *The complete education gives one not only power of concentration,*
> *but worthy objectives upon which to concentrate."*[104]
>
> —Dr. Martin Luther King, Jr., American civil rights leader, 1929–1968

In fall 2010, President Barack Obama charged the Bioethics Commission with overseeing a fact-finding historical review of research conducted and supported by the U.S. Public Health Service in Guatemala in the 1940s that involved deliberately exposing human subjects to certain sexually transmitted diseases without their consent. Records of this research, which involved vulnerable populations, including prisoners and hospitalized psychiatric patients, were discovered in 2003. When the discovery was made public in 2010, the U.S. Government responded swiftly to the revelation with apologies to the Guatemalan government and its people.[105]

In addition to the fact-finding investigation, the President charged the Bioethics Commission with reviewing contemporary human subjects research protections to determine if they are adequate to safeguard the health and wellbeing of human participants in research. To answer the charge, the Commission conducted a thorough historical review, examining thousands of documents to learn the details of the 1940s research; it conducted four public meetings in 1 year and invited experts from diverse subject areas. This work highlighted numerous topics in professional and research ethics, both of which served to educate both the public and the research community.

After the release of its report, *"Ethically Impossible" STD Research in Guatemala from 1946 to 1948,* and a companion report, *Moral Science: Protecting Participants in Human Subjects Research*, the Bioethics Commission released eight educational modules to accompany the reports, including a study guide companion to the report, which was later translated into Spanish.[106]

Regardless of whether we are aware of it, bioethics affects us all. This is the single most salient reason that ethics education and ethics literacy are essential for guiding both individuals and deliberative bodies. As individuals, we have no alternative but to navigate an increasingly complex health care system for ourselves and our loved ones. As voters, taxpayers, and community members, we must decide what communal values should guide policy on fundamental questions of birth and death, health, and wellbeing—or these will be decided for us. As scientists, clinicians, and lawyers, to fulfill our professional obligations, we must resolve dilemmas, understand the obligations of our professions, and attend to the broader social impacts of our work. In each of these roles, the ability to recognize, articulate, and resolve ethical challenges is absolutely essential.

National bioethics bodies like ours can accept an increasingly important role by encouraging and supporting bioethics education. This Bioethics Commission has strived to fulfill this role in several ways. We have developed educational materials related to our reports to reach diverse audiences. We participate in deliberation and learn details of particular topics to gain a deeper understanding of how ethics principles we have learned throughout our lives, both personally and professionally, should be applied to the open questions we face as a federal commission. In modeling this educational component of deliberative democracy, we aim to encourage future generations of bioethicists, scientists, health care providers, other professionals, and the public at large to become informed and make reasoned decisions in this pluralistic society. As the Bioethics Commission nears the end of its tenure, we encourage future bioethics advisory bodies to continue to fulfill this role, as bodies before us have done.

Bioethics education cannot be crafted and conducted solely at the national level. We also need to build a foundation of ethical reasoning at all levels of society. Ethics education is a multilevel and intergenerational process of building ethics literacy: a basic understanding of ethics concepts and language that can serve as the bedrock of civil discourse and of individual and collective decision making. Schools from pre-kindergarten to professional training programs can and should incorporate ethics education into their curricula to help build the ethics literacy that will enable us to reason through complex bioethical problems we all will face. Ethics education can raise the population's ethics and scientific literacy and can help prepare everyone for the difficult conversations and decisions that bioethics presents.

We focus here on ethics education primarily in bioethics for two reasons. First, bioethics is the area in which we can deploy our Commission's expertise to greatest effect. Second, bioethical concerns permeate our culture, society, and lifespan. They concern matters of life and death and deeply held personal values. They raise fundamental questions of how we should coexist and what we owe one another as fellow humans. Bioethics requires us to reason and deliberate together, and for that, we all need an understanding of ethics to articulate and justify our beliefs, understand how our values intersect with those of our fellow community members, and provide the basis for collective decision making on matters of common concern.

Throughout its tenure, the Bioethics Commission has emphasized the societal importance of bioethics education. It has recommended improving ethics education for health, science, and technology students and professionals, as well as consumers of health services and technologies. The Bioethics Commission's commitment to strengthening educational efforts to promote greater ethics literacy is demonstrated by its numerous recommendations across reports for increasing the depth and breadth of bioethics education. Building on this commitment and on current attention to national education policy after the passage of the Every Student Succeeds Act in 2015, the Bioethics Commission takes this opportunity to reinvigorate a national discussion about ethics education and our collective responsibility for ensuring that our society is prepared to make informed and justifiable decisions about morally complex aspects of science, technology, and health policy.[107]

This section describes how ethics education can be infused throughout all levels of education, from primary school through professional and postgraduate training. It also addresses how learning about moral topics outside traditional learning settings, including as community members, plays an important role in creating an informed and engaged public. It then considers some of the obstacles to implementing ethics education and how these might be overcome.

* * *

Ethics education encompasses broad instructional practices and experiences that develop one's ability to make and act on considered moral judgments. To facilitate clarity, three related but distinct concepts should be distinguished: *education of bioethicists, bioethics education,* and the broader notion of *ethics education.*

Education of Bioethicists

Education of bioethicists is the process of educating someone to enter the field of bioethics. Bioethics is a broad interdisciplinary set of practices that includes academic inquiry, policy analysis, and practical guidance relating to science, technology, and health topics. Because no single disciplinary path exists for entering this field—and this diversity is a key strength—professionals who consider themselves bioethicists often have their primary training in one field (e.g., law, medicine, nursing, science, or philosophy) and additional formal or informal training in ethics or bioethics. This notion of *dual competence* has been a hallmark of those educated in bioethics since the inception of the field.[108]

Since the early 2000s, the opportunity for formal bioethics training—in the form of post-baccalaureate certificates and master's degrees—has increased substantially, in part because of growth in the number of programs in these areas offered by universities and other tertiary institutions.[109] This trend adds to the complexity of longstanding and ongoing discourse about the identity and strength of bioethics as an interdisciplinary field.[110] Although bioethicists play a principal role in certain professional settings, the majority of the population will face bioethical challenges throughout their lives and need skills to work through them.

> "Although bioethics is central to the education of health care professionals, its reach should be much broader. Health care is important to all members of society, and therefore bioethics should be a concern of every citizen. Every citizen should give thought to whether they want to be an organ donor, and to what kind of care they want to receive at the end of life. It is, therefore, our responsibility to ensure that all members of society understand the importance of bioethics and that we provide opportunities for reflection on these issues."
>
> Lehmann, L., Director, Center for Bioethics, Brigham and Women's Hospital; Associate Professor of Medicine and Medical Ethics, Harvard Medical School; Associate Professor of Health Policy and Management, Harvard School of Public Health. (2014). Deliberation and Bioethics Education: Overview. Presentation to the Bioethics Commission, November 6. Retrieved March 22, 2016 from http://bioethics.gov/node/4321.

Bioethics Education

Bioethics education encompasses efforts to engage students in various science, technology, and health-related contexts that include complex ethical, social, and legal dimensions. One key purpose of bioethics education is preparing individuals for making decisions about their own health and that of others.[111]

Bioethics education fosters skills that will help students confront decisions that they will inevitably face—how to contend with a difficult medical diagnosis, what aspects to consider when making treatment decisions, how to be a good caregiver, and how to make plans for the end of life. We can make better decisions when we develop and use skills to recognize, articulate, and consider the ethical dimensions of how we ought to proceed. Learning these skills is a life-long process requiring foundational skills in ethics; opportunities to apply these skills are abundant in personal and professional life.

Both formal and informal bioethics education is instrumental to improving public understanding of the ethical dimensions of emerging technologies, human subjects research, clinical decision making, public health emergencies, advances in neuroscience, and more. Bioethics education helps to build the scientific and ethics literacy individuals need for understanding the implications of these complex matters for their own life as well as that of their loved ones and their communities.

Ethics Education

"A serious argument can be made that, while we teach American school children multiple materials, largely because we always have, we fail to teach them content that is vital to full participation in the life of contemporary democracy."

Steiner, D., Executive Director, Johns Hopkins Institute for Education Policy; Professor, School of Education, Johns Hopkins University. (2015). Implementing Innovations in Ethics Education. Presentation to the Bioethics Commission, November 17. Retrieved March 23, 2016 from http://bioethics.gov/node/5358.

Everyone, including those training to be bioethics professionals and those who might encounter a bioethical challenge during their lifetime, needs a foundation of general ethics education on which to build more specific bioethical moral reasoning. Ethics education fosters the ability to identify, articulate, and act upon justified moral positions. It develops skills of critical and practical reasoning through which students learn to question, strengthen, inform, and enrich their own positions in light of others' perspectives. Ethical analysis and reasoning is often coupled with problem-solving and active learning, enabling students to challenge, reflect on, and learn how to enact and live up to their professed values. Ethics requires that students understand how and why their views resemble or differ from others' views. This aspect of ethics education intersects with the values and skills of democratic deliberation, described in the previous chapter, including mutual respect and public spiritedness.

Integration of ethics education into other classroom activities has long been part of educational discourse in the United States. In 1749, Benjamin Franklin recommended moral teaching for Pennsylvania's youth, proposing that history lessons can be used to build moral character, foster aesthetic appreciation, and instill a sense of public spirit, among other aims.[112] Ethics education can be integrated into existing curricula by introducing subject-relevant ethical dilemmas or challenges into classes in which they are likely to arise (e.g., the sciences, history, social studies, economics, or media studies). Concrete examples and problem-based learning help to ground ethics discussions in their practical implications that connect to students' current and future experiences. Understanding complex science topics, for example, is facilitated by the critical interpretation skills and intellectual curiosity fostered by ethical analysis, and ethics can even "whet students' appetites" for science, increasing interest among students who might otherwise perceive science as uninteresting or irrelevant.[113] Moreover, both ethics and science are necessary for arriving at the best solutions to complex problems in scientific practice and policy. Well-reasoned arguments for action must be guided by the best available evidence; in turn, attaining high standards in ethical scientific practice requires honing skills in reflection, analysis, and decision making.

Ethics Education Across the Lifespan

Ethics education should start early, building a foundation for ongoing learning. Early ethics education provides a base on which to build skills to engage with the ethical dimensions of subjects taught in postsecondary school, as well as ethical matters in specific professions. In addition, ethics education at different stages of life helps individuals confront ethical choices as individuals, family and community members, and professionals.

Ethics education can and should be incorporated throughout education, from curricula

"[T]o prepare students for modern life, we need to teach in a way that cuts across disciplinary boundaries to offer skills and resources that transfer across what is all too often a divide between the classroom and life and learning and career outside of school.... The interdisciplinary study of bioethics provides a very natural way for teachers to reach across disciplines, to engage their students in complex and real issues, to provide relevant learning and research opportunities around topics of contemporary concern."

Bishop, L., Head of Academic Programs, Kennedy Institute of Ethics, Georgetown University. (2015). Implementing Innovations in Ethics Education. Presentation to the Bioethics Commission, November 17. Retrieved March 23, 2016 from http://bioethics.gov/node/5358.

in primary school through secondary school, to undergraduate coursework, graduate school, and professional training programs. Ethics education is best when it builds on itself over time. To build ethics literacy, broad-based ethics education must start early, before students begin to track into more specialized interests and careers. Over time, ethics education should become more targeted, and provide preparation for the particular challenges that health, science, and technology professionals are likely to face.

> "[S]tart early to raise ethical literacy… All of us need skills to help us resolve ethical issues, whether we are a plumber or a physician or a scientist…[we will need these skills if] we become a surrogate decision maker, [and] many of us will."
>
> Lee, L.M., Executive Director, Presidential Commission for the Study of Bioethical Issues. (2015). Roundtable Discussion. Presentation to the Bioethics Commission, September 2. Retrieved March 23, 2016 from http://bioethics.gov/node/5269.

The nature and content of ethics education depend on context. With younger students, ethics education might consist of a broad base of pedagogy about basic moral principles by using different age-appropriate methods to encourage children to start thinking about morality and ethics and by using examples they might encounter during their lifetime. In undergraduate courses, discussion and instruction on ethical and social issues might be tied more closely to specific subjects—for example, a molecular biology class might consider the ethics of stem cell research. In graduate or professional school, ethics training can be tailored to particular issues that professionals in that field are likely to encounter. Mentoring, case discussions, and ethics consultations are opportunities for continuing ethics education for professionals throughout their careers. At the community level, less formal ethics education can occur through discussion forums or opportunities to contribute to local ethics review boards or institutional ethics committees. Ethics education is most engaging when it addresses situations relevant to an individual's immediate or near-future contexts.[114] The following sections describe examples of ethics education programs at different levels and educational settings.

Outside the Classroom

Broadly understood, education encompasses all features of society that inspire learning and self-realization.[115] On this broad view, as John Stuart Mill stated, education is "[w]hatever helps to shape the human being; to make the individual what he is, or hinder him from being what he is not…"[116] In the context of institutions such as schools, colleges, and universities, education takes on a more specific meaning, conveying what "each generation purposely gives to those who are to be its successors, in order to qualify them for at least keeping up, and if possible for raising, the level of improvement which has been attained."[117] Mill's remarks point out the connections between education, ethics, and identity, highlighting the importance of both kinds of ethics education.

Moral insights are gained from experiences of all kinds: the circumstances we encounter, the challenges we face, and the choices we make. Many individuals and diverse social and cultural institutions play crucial roles in broad ethics education. Relationships of all kinds are important teachers, even if moral instruction is not their main purpose. Families, for one, are a central source of learning about values, especially early in life as loved ones communicate and instill distinct familial values throughout childhood and into adolescence. Parenthood is also educational, providing individuals with new insights that lead them to question, develop, and understand their parental obligations. Relationships can spark knowledge relevant to moral development throughout adolescence and adulthood, revealing an individual's own capacity for love, patience, growth, compassion, and reciprocity.

Communities are also important sources of values, often linking more formal articulations of values and principles to individual and community identities. In a pluralistic society, individuals participate in and seek out shared ways of life, sometimes strengthening old ties and sometimes forming new ones. From the implicit messages within the aphorisms passed on through generations to the explicit moral education of religious communities, these traditions reflect the diversity of ways we learn to live up to our values in practice. By participating in and forming communities, instilling character, and fostering habits, individuals learn to enact their values in deeds as well as words.

Drawing from complex and varied sources of moral life, a broad ethics education does not contradict the more focused goals found in traditional learning settings. On the contrary, each influences the other. Whether inside or outside the walls of a classroom, different forms of education enrich our moral development.

Primary School

Ethics education must start early to prepare a strong foundation on which to build the ethics skills one needs in adult life, and to help children develop into better world citizens as they mature. Teaching ethics to adults or professionals as a starting point is inconsistent with evidence of how education and learning builds throughout time and with our understanding of moral development. Just as we would not expect to develop math skills in an engineer or an accountant by starting with calculus, similarly, we cannot expect to develop ethics literacy unless we build an early foundation starting with the basics. Studies indicate that children as young as 2 years are capable of engaging with critical reasoning in moral judgment and can begin to distinguish between moral rules and social conventions as early as preschool.[118] In early education, we can also start to build moral character, including the formation of moral sensitivity, moral identity, and lasting habits, all of which are important for future ethical decision making.

An innovative example of ethics education in primary school is a program developed for students in New South Wales, Australia.[119] The curriculum for the program is organized around age-appropriate questions, scenarios, and case studies that encourage students to think for themselves. The youngest children, for example, consider such questions as whether telling others a friend's secret is okay or whether being frustrated with someone justifies physically hurting that individual. Older children consider more complex questions for example, whether being fair means giving everyone in the group an equal share or what counts as cheating. Often the questions are closely related to a child's everyday experiences.[120] The program emphasizes both "sequential and spiral" learning, meaning the curriculum revisits the questions through progressively more detailed engagement as the children get older and advance through the program.[121] Because the classes are led by volunteers from the community, including parents and grandparents, the program also makes a distinctive contribution to broader public ethics education and ethics literacy.

The United States does not have national requirements for ethics education in schools. Decisions about curricular content and resources for implementation of content are under the purview of state and local

> "Our aim is to have children think for themselves about, for example, the extent to which the intention of the agent is important when judging rightness or wrongness of, say, breaking a promise. We want children to think about whether we need to take the circumstances into account when deciding whether a particular act of lying is wrong. We want them to think carefully about their relationships with their friends and to consider whether they care about their friends for their friends' own sakes or whether they might be simply using their friends for their own ends, and if they are, whether that's okay. And we want them to think about how important it is to be a good person, to live a good life and, if it is important, what character traits we need to develop in pursuit of this goal."
>
> Knight, S., Curriculum Author, Primary Ethics Limited Australia. (2015). Ethical and Deliberative Skills across the Lifespan. Presentation to the Bioethics Commission, September 2. Retrieved March 23, 2016 from http://bioethics.gov/node/5267.

governments. Character.org, a national nonprofit organization, supports character development programs in schools, providing leadership and resources to "develop ethical citizens committed to building a just and caring world."[122] Their program supports school systems and administrators in any district or state, and includes teacher training and lesson plans for elementary and secondary educators. Approximately 5,000 U.S. schools and districts, representing half a million students, have participated in the program since it began in 1998.[123]

Secondary School

After we have built a foundation of ethics education by developing character and moral identity among young children, we continue to cultivate moral development in the higher grades. By high school, students' understanding of morality and their own values start to solidify. High school is an opportune time to incorporate ethics education and discussion into existing topic-based classes—high school teachers can start to incorporate ethical questions into existing curricula and to apply ethical reasoning to specific topics and problems regarding class content. In secondary school biology, chemistry, social studies, history, and other subjects, teachers can incorporate ethical questions or problems and exercises with ethical dimensions. Students can apply ethical decision-making skills, engage in self-reflection and discussion among peers, and begin to understand bioethics concepts.

Some mistakenly assume that bioethics education should be provided to high-achieving students only.[124] Previous research on mathematics education has demonstrated that students of higher socioeconomic status have more opportunity to learn than students of lower socioeconomic status.[125] Assuming this trend also exists in science education, bioethics education—when integrated into science classes—might exacerbate these inequities. Professional development for teachers of all subjects at all levels can be designed to anticipate and confront these dynamics so that student opportunities for engagement are more justly distributed. Fair distribution of these types of educational opportunities is especially important because evidence indicates that education in civic engagement might also promote student achievement in other areas, including attainment of higher levels of education.[126]

Multiple efforts have been made to implement bioethics education at the high school level in the United States. In 1990, The Hastings Center, the New Jersey Science Education Leadership Association (then the New Jersey Science Supervisors Association), and Roche Pharmaceuticals (then Hoffman-La Roche) published a teaching resource to help high school science teachers in New Jersey incorporate bioethics concepts into their classrooms.[127] The resource contained case studies, lesson plans, and teaching strategies on such topics as genetics and environmental responsibility.[128] In the Northern Valley Regional High School District in Bergen County, New Jersey, project leaders provided a 3-day in-service program to train teachers on using the supplement.[129] More recently, the Kennedy Institute of Ethics at Georgetown University developed a high school bioethics curriculum to equip teachers with classroom materials that can be integrated into existing curricula.[130] The National Institutes of Health *Exploring Bioethics* curricular supplement provides science teachers with six classroom modules and learning activities that address bioethics considerations associated with specific topics, ranging from "Balancing Individual and Community Claims: Establishing State Vaccination Policies" to "Modifying the Natural World: Human Responsibilities Toward Animals."[131]

In programs like these, teacher training and support is essential. Teachers face multiple challenges when incorporating ethics into high school classrooms. By high school, students begin to individuate from their parents, developing their own values and perspectives. They develop curiosity about the world and morality. Teachers must be prepared to consider tough questions without offending parents or school administrators, control potentially heated classroom discussions, and provide tools to help students differentiate between facts, opinions, values, and ethical perspectives. Support for teachers through these programs has included professional development workshops, course materials to structure classroom discussions, and viable solutions to challenges related to teaching ethics.[132]

"[I]n terms of creating safe space for students to have these kinds of discussions, we first have to care about helping the teachers be prepared, and that's not a trivial task because teacher preparation, as everybody knows, is very different across different places and they have a lot on their plates."

Grady, C., Chief, Department of Bioethics, National Institutes of Health (NIH) Clinical Center; Senior Research Fellow, Kennedy Institute of Ethics, Georgetown University. (2015). Member Discussion, November 17. Retrieved March 23, 2016 from http://bioethics. gov/node/5357.

Structured deliberative activities, developed by Diana Hess, use deliberative methods to teach controversial topics—including bioethical concepts—in high school settings. These activities involve structured discussions that focus on specific, intentionally chosen problems with the students placed at the fore of the discussion rather than the teacher. Although consensus is not required at the end of these activities, they are structured to foster high-quality deliberation in which students engage each other's views respectfully rather than amplify disagreement. Hess offers three specific activity models that can be effective in teaching deliberation involving controversial topics.

The first activity is the "Town Meeting Model."[133] Students assume the roles, interests, and beliefs of actors and stakeholders in a town meeting on a public policy discussion. Background material tailored for each role is studied in preparation for the meeting. During the meeting, students drive the discussion, and the teacher serves as moderator, calling on students and intervening infrequently to redirect the conversation or pose a pointed question to spark new insights. Led by the teacher, the students debrief after the activity, reflecting on what went well and what went poorly.[134]

The second activity is the "Seminar Model."[135] In this activity, discussion centers on a specific text. The purpose of limiting the discussion to one text is to develop a deeper understanding of the issues and arguments presented in the text. In this text-based seminar, students must refer back to the text to provide evidence for their arguments. They must consider multiple perspectives and strive to present all arguments in their best light. The teacher poses questions to facilitate discussion and might raise and defend a minority viewpoint to avoid a premature consensus.[136]

The third activity is the "Public Issues Discussion Model."[137] In this activity, the teacher splits the class into smaller discussion groups to address controversial topics. Before the activity, students are taught about methods of effective and respectful discussion and must strive to implement them in the subsequent activity. The teacher mostly observes the discussions, assessing students on their ability to engage in reasoned and respectful discussion. Occasionally, the teacher might challenge the students' analysis or invite a minority view to deepen the deliberations.[138]

These are promising models because they align "theory and practice, teaching *for* and *with* discussion."[139] That is, these activities impart knowledge and develop skills in high-quality discussion. In this way, these activities serve as mechanisms both for learning about specific concepts and as forums for developing skills for respectful democratic deliberation.

Postsecondary School

After high school, students' environments change substantially. Many students are living away from home for the first time. College can expose students to individuals with many different backgrounds, values, and perspectives. After building a strong base of moral character and ethical reasoning skills in primary school and applying those skills to specific topics in secondary school, ethics education in college offers further opportunity to continue to apply and specify. In undergraduate education, students start to specialize their learning, choosing tracks and majors. Ethics education in college courses can start to teach students how to identify, confront, and resolve ethical dilemmas they will encounter as professionals. The college classroom environment, with greater diversity of peers and perspectives, will help students articulate their values and refine their ethics in relation to the broader world.

Bioethics education has been integrated across undergraduate curricula in different ways. For example, the Kennedy Institute of Ethics has implemented several ethics education initiatives at Georgetown University that demonstrate the diverse opportunities for instructors to collaborate in developing interdisciplinary learning opportunities related to ethics.[140] Through the *Conversations in Bioethics* series, students and classes study a bioethics topic during the fall semester. In the spring semester, speakers with relevant expertise or experience are invited to present to the entire student body, opening up campus-wide conversations. The institute has also pioneered *Ethics Lab*, where students from different majors grapple with ethics in a practical way by creating products to address complex problems with both scientific and ethical dimensions.[141]

Online teaching has also been used to increase access to bioethics education, presenting the opportunity to reach a large and diverse group of learners. The Kennedy Institute's bioethics massive open online course (MOOC), Introduction to Bioethics, is open to students worldwide, and during 2015, included 5,000 participants.[142] The cultural exposure that college can bring— transporting students to different environments where they are confronted with diverse peers—can be magnified in the MOOC setting. On the Internet, an even more diverse set of backgrounds, attitudes, and beliefs exists. Students learning about ethics in the MOOC context learn how to conduct ethical decision making and articulate ethical beliefs in a broader context.

Team teaching is a commonly used instructional approach to ethics education at the postsecondary level.[143] Mirroring the notion of dual competence, the goal of team teaching is to integrate different disciplines, for example ethics and law or ethics and public health, bringing them to bear on complex problems. Foresight and careful planning is needed to overcome obstacles that might make team-teaching difficult, including cost, administrative obstacles, and logistical challenges.[144]

Another edifying and engaging opportunity for college students to learn ethics is the extracurricular Intercollegiate Ethics Bowl, which celebrated its 20th year in 2016. Ethics Bowl teams comprise interested students with diverse backgrounds and majors and one or more faculty sponsors. Teams deliberate, reach consensus, and present their perspectives on cases with challenging ethical dimensions. The teams reason their way to an answer, present their responses to a panel of judges, and respond to follow-up questions that challenge their application of ethical reasoning to the case. Competing teams comment on one another's presentations. After both teams complete this process, the judges evaluate the teams' performance in four categories: intelligibility, depth, focus, and judgment. The Ethics Bowl provides unique educational benefits, helping students develop a framework for ethical reasoning and understanding about a broad range of issues. It also fosters an appreciation for "viewing from the inside other ethical positions besides those with which a person agrees."[145]

Unlike classroom discussion, which tends to be instructor-driven and lacks direct engagement between students' viewpoints, the Ethics Bowl requires students to deliberate within their teams and present a unified response despite likely disagreement among team members. The consensus-building aspect of the activity ensures that "[e]ither differences of opinion narrow with further discussion, or, if not, team members nonetheless develop a clearer understanding of each other's positions."[146] The ability to listen to and appreciate the force of opposing viewpoints is integral to effective deliberation and ethical understanding of complex, controversial topics about which reasonable people can genuinely disagree.[147] Although the activity covers a range of academic, professional, and personal subjects, bioethics topics are included as well.[148] A national undergraduate Bioethics Bowl—following the same format as other Ethics Bowls but exclusively featuring cases and questions about bioethics topics—is held annually.[149]

The Intercollegiate Ethics Bowl requires teams to qualify for the highest levels of competition.[150] Although this tiered structure restricts the number of teams that can compete for the championship, the educational impact of the Ethics Bowl is not limited to those at the highest competition levels. For example, the Illinois Institute of Technology's Intercollegiate Ethics Bowl team—which has involved students from a variety of majors (e.g., architecture, business, and biomedical engineering)—is embedded in a student organization that hosts multiple campus events to engage students in conversations about ethics.[151]

Professional and Graduate School

Ethics education becomes even more applied and specific in professional and graduate school. In addition to concepts learned in a classroom setting, graduate students and professionals frequently need to address real-world

"Anecdotally what I have seen is an incredible hunger for [communications training] among the generation of scientists that are coming up through the system now. At the Graduate Program in Science Writing—that has always been for journalists—there has been an enormous uptick in science Ph.D. students who want to enroll in that program simultaneously...."

Mnookin, S., Associate Director, MIT Graduate Program in Science Writing. (2015). Fluency in Science and Ethics. Presentation to the Bioethics Commission, September 2. Retrieved March 24, 2016 from http://bioethics.gov/node/5266.

problems. They need skills to identify and articulate the ethical dimensions of their work, to deliberate with colleagues and others, and to implement and evaluate solutions.

Professional training and development can—and sometimes does—introduce tailored curricula that explore ethics topics in context, situating ethical questions in settings that resemble those that professionals will encounter in research, medicine, engineering, or business. Applied and contextual learning experiences can be created for professionals with the goal of developing the critical reasoning skills and desired habits of mind that are reflective of dedicated and thoughtful experts and leaders.[152]

Professional degrees—including the sciences, medicine, nursing, public health, engineering, journalism, and business—often include ethics coursework as a requirement or option. A few medical schools incorporated the humanities and human values into their curricula as early as the 1960s, and more followed in the 1970s as medical progress galvanized public interest in ethical questions.[153] A 2004 survey revealed that 78% of medical schools integrated ethics into preclinical courses.[154] Case-based discussion is the most common pedagogical approach to medical ethics education and is often combined with other approaches, including team teaching, small-group article discussions, reflective writing media presentations, and role-playing.[155]

"The first goal [of bioethics education in nursing] is to stimulate students to critically reflect upon and question the values, beliefs, and assumptions that they bring to clinical practice in an atmosphere that supports and respects diversity of intellectual thought, cultural paradigms, and respect for persons."

Ulrich, C., Associate Professor of Bioethics in Nursing, University of Pennsylvania School of Nursing. (2015). Goals of and Approaches to Bioethics Education. Presentation to the Bioethics Commission, May 27. Retrieved March 24, 2016 from http://bioethics.gov/node/4945.

Bioethics education programs are crucial, albeit not always required, in public health and nursing training. Although public health professionals report facing ethical challenges, only half of accredited schools of public health require any ethics courses.[156] A survey of practicing nurses indicated that, without such training, nurses are less likely to take action or seek assistance with an ethical problem and are more vulnerable to moral distress—distress arising from the tension between what is being done and what one thinks should be done.[157]

Advanced training in the natural sciences, including in biomedical research, typically includes some ethics education through responsible conduct of research training. However, such training has been perceived to emphasize regulatory compliance over scientists' abilities to reflect on and contend with the ethical and social challenges arising in their work.[158] Enabling scientists to explore the ethical and social implications of their work is an important, yet frequently overlooked, responsibility for institutions of higher education in the United States.[159] Expanded curricula should address dynamics that the Bioethics Commission has focused on in previous reports, for example, the hype that often accompanies research results.[160]

Mentoring of professional students is an important mechanism for communicating the norms, expectations, and obligations of a profession. Many assume that most character formation is complete by the time students reach graduate school. However, graduate and career training inevitably involve acculturation to the dominant professional norms. Professional schools should attend to fostering professional virtues such as trustworthiness and compassion and try to counter institutional environments that erode students' ideals.[161] Evidence suggests that mentoring can influence students toward or away from unethical practices.[162] To foster virtue and counter negative influences, certain approaches emphasize that graduate-level ethics education must bridge theory and practice, connecting professionalism to identity formation.[163] Given its relation to identity, ongoing ethics education involves expanding on earlier moral lessons, drawing on exemplars and insights from both inside and outside the classroom (Figure 4).

Adult Bioethics Education in Public and Private Life

Bioethics education continues beyond formal education and professional training. A broad base in ethics education provides a solid foundation on which to build abilities for engaging with life's ethical dimensions in postsecondary school, including highly contextual ethical concerns in the professions.

FIGURE 4

ETHICS EDUCATION ACROSS THE LIFESPAN

PROFESSIONAL AND GRADUATE SCHOOL
Applying to situations encountered in the profession

Example: Identify and articulate ethical dimensions of field-specific problems, develop solutions

POSTSECONDARY SCHOOL
Enhancing skills to confront and resolve ethical dilemmas in specific fields

Example: Refine ethical arguments using relevant texts, draw from examples in given field of study, develop ethics decision-making skills

SECONDARY SCHOOL
Developing character and moral identity

Example: Develop personal views on ethical issues raised in class, discuss and defend those views with peers

PRIMARY SCHOOL
Forming the foundations of moral development, simple maxims

Example: Learn simple lessons about sharing, non-violence, etc. through age-appropriate examples

Ethics education starts with a broad foundation in primary school, cultivating character and moral reasoning. As students get older, ethics education builds on the foundation, becoming more specific and tailored to students' career trajectories, professional lives, and community membership.

In addition, ethics education throughout life prepares individuals to address ethical choices in their lives both as private individuals and as members of their communities. Most of us have or will confront bioethical questions about what we should do in the face of difficult health-related decisions for ourselves or our loved ones. As our population ages, questions about living and dying well will become more than hypothetical. As members of communities, we are often called upon to help make decisions about the public good and allocation of limited resources. We participate in public decision making about bioethics and health policies in various ways—when we vote, pay taxes, write or email public officials, and attend public meetings. Even for adults who do not continue their education past secondary or postsecondary levels, ethics literacy and an understanding of values and moral reasoning are necessary both for private and public ethical decision making.

One public effort in bioethics education implemented in Australia, the European Union, and North America is the death café, a community-based forum intended to help individuals understand their preferences and options at the end of life and overcome reluctance to think about or discuss death.[164] In addition to real-time gatherings such as death cafés, other materials are available for free online to help adults make bioethical decisions. The Bioethics Commission's educational materials include a set of primers for the public. These "Conversation Series" materials provide patients, research participants, and consumers with a guide to incidental findings, the focus of the 2013 report, *Anticipate and Communicate: Ethical Management of Incidental and Secondary Findings in the Clinical, Research, and Direct-to-Consumer Contexts.*

"[A] lot of [ethics education], I think, is getting at the kind of subtle, nuanced, rich language that is ethical language because it helps you to interpret what you're seeing and that helps set the stage for how to think about it. So an example might be…the difference between discrimination and subordination. That's powerful to people because it lets them name a reality that they might not otherwise have words for."

Little, M., Director, Kennedy Institute of Ethics; Professor of Philosophy, Georgetown University. (2015). Goals of and Approaches to Bioethics Education. Presentation to the Bioethics Commission, May 27. Retrieved March 24, 2016 from http://bioethics.gov/node/4945.

These guides help individuals understand key ethical considerations related to incidental findings and clinical, research, and direct-to-consumer testing. For patients and participants, they help determine what questions should be asked during a visit with a clinician or to the research team to prepare for the findings.

Throughout adulthood, an individual has many opportunities to engage with and learn about bioethics topics. Local universities and community colleges offer lifelong learning and continuing education opportunities. Short courses often address such topics as surveys of ethics and law in medicine and aging with dignity. Community organizations and churches also host classes, talks, and discussions engaging different topics such as ethics and religious teachings; pressing issues in current events; surveys of world religions; and ethical implications of advances in health, science, and technology. Adult learning opportunities provide for ongoing engagement with, and sometimes new exposure to, moral traditions and communities. In addition, these forms of learning offer much-needed guided exposure to the constantly changing technologic landscape of modern society, and such learning opportunities frequently attend to adults' shifting needs and interests through all of life's stages.

Advocacy organizations focused on specific conditions also can serve as an educational resource for ethical concerns that arise among affected individuals. For example, the Alzheimer's Association provides educational information for surrogate decision makers to help them make choices for those with the disease regarding research participation.[165] The Alzheimer's Association also has created a list of resources for individuals with dementia and their families addressing rapidly changing scientific advances and ethical complexities surrounding Alzheimer's disease and dementia.[166]

A 2000 AARP survey indicated that keeping up with "what's going on in the world" and seeking "spiritual or personal growth" were top motivations for interest in learning among adults age 50 years and over.[167] Especially relevant to ethics education, respondents also cited desires to help, understand, and get along better with others.[168] Importantly, a large portion of surveyed adults also indicated they had experienced a personal illness, the illness or death of a family member, or becoming a caregiver for an older family member during the previous year.[169] These findings provide evidence that encouraging bioethics education for adult learners can be especially important.

Obstacles and Potential Solutions

Integrating ethics into education at all levels is a promising model for increasing ethics literacy and teaching students how to examine the subjects they are studying through the lens of ethics.[170] Yet teachers might be reluctant to introduce ethical considerations into the classroom. This reluctance can pose serious challenges to integrating ethics education into existing educational structures, but these challenges can be overcome. This section describes some of those obstacles that lead to reluctance, which can include lack of training, concern from parents or administrators about indoctrination, and logistical and practical challenges. It then provides some methods for addressing and attenuating these obstacles.

The first and perhaps most substantial obstacle is lack of teacher training or preparation. Teachers might think that teaching or leading a discussion on an ethics topic requires expertise that they lack, or they might believe that teaching the ethical aspects of a subject like science is not their responsibility and should be reserved for a class dedicated to bioethics.[171] Training materials and guides have been developed to help teachers understand and prepare for teaching ethics topics as part of their existing curricula.

Training and support can address teachers' concerns that they will lose control of their classrooms if challenging or controversial ethics topics arise. The increasingly polarized political and social climate makes many topics with ethical dimensions seem untouchable. Teachers are worried that classroom discussions will become disorderly.

Some scholars argue that, instead of abandoning political discussion and deliberative democracy because of polarization, we must instead embrace it.[172] Discussions with other teachers and experts about strategies and pedagogical techniques can help teachers develop skills in managing and promoting discussions of ethical issues in their classrooms. For example, the Northwest Association for Biomedical Research, a body that promotes public understanding of biomedical research and its ethical conduct, has developed resources for training and supporting teachers when integrating ethics topics into science classrooms.[173] These resources, available on their website, include curricula that describe relevant scientific and ethical issues on specific topics (e.g., human immunodeficiency virus vaccines) and an *Ethics Primer*, which describes ethical theories, decision-making frameworks, and classroom strategies.[174] Teachers can also participate in annual workshops designed for practicing strategies outlined in the primer and developing lesson plans and case studies.[175]

Another resource for teachers is the free online National Institutes of Health bioethics curriculum material. *Exploring Bioethics*, mentioned previously, is a curricular supplement for biology classes in grades 9–12 created to provide an opportunity for students to address complex bioethics topics and develop critical thinking and problem-solving skills. These teaching materials include information for instructors about handling common challenges in teaching bioethics which is useful at all educational levels.[176]

Ethics education initiatives should be developed and implemented in accordance with the best available evidence about what works, making ongoing research and evaluation essential for success. Research and evaluation can take different forms, from surveys conducted by the teacher to large independent studies. Teachers should set goals for what each class or program is attempting to achieve so that they can more easily assess their success. Evidence gathered can then be used to design more effective future classes. For example, the Romanell Report on medical ethics education, released in 2015, identified ways of evaluating ethics education, including self-assessment, reflective practice, evaluation in changes of attitudes, performance portfolios, examinations that assess knowledge, clinical evaluation exercises, objective structured clinical examinations, and small-group discussions with feedback.[177] Directors of ethics courses in medical schools also have used different methods for assessing medical students' ethical learning, including class participation, examinations, papers, case analyses, behaviors, and journals.[178]

Robust evaluation often requires attention to both short- and long-term outcomes.[179] Immediate pre- and post-intervention surveys and assessments are a common way of evaluating a particular teaching method, an assignment, grasp of student material or attainment of a skill set, as well as the overall influence of a course. Other types of research focused on long-term outcomes include periodic follow-up surveys or interviews. Comprehensive programs—rather than teaching approaches or individual courses—can use measures such as enrollment in a particular major or attendance at conferences to assess interest.[180]

"[Evaluation] can really help give us feedback about what we're doing well and maybe to help us tweak our goals and make sure that we're meeting them.... [I]t can also, then, provide accountability to our stakeholders, to ourselves—to see if we are meeting our goals—and to our constituencies, our funders, our participants."

Ripple, C. Associate Director for Education Research and Engagement, Duke University Social Science Research Institute. (2015). Fostering and Measuring Success in Ethics and Deliberation. Presentation to the Bioethics Commission, September 2. Retrieved January 22, 2016 from http://bioethics.gov/node/5268.

A second obstacle to infusing ethics across the curriculum is resistance from administrators or parents, some of whom believe that ethics is subjective, that younger students are incapable of high-level reasoning or deliberation, or that ethics education imposes particular values on students—values that might not match their own.[181] On the contrary, ethics education teaches students *how* to think, not *what* to think. It involves helping students understand different perspectives and schools of thought and to develop analytic and respectful deliberative skills that help them avoid an uncritical acceptance of values. One purpose of ethics education is to encourage students to understand their own views, recognizing that a classroom discussion might be the first time that they think carefully and critically about a particular topic.[182] Moreover, discussion of an ethical question might expose students to a broader range of views and values than they have previously encountered, helping them consider the matter from a new perspective.

"Another problem is that the public often doesn't want students to hear points of view that are different than their own. Parents, in particular, sometimes believe that it's important that schools…perfectly reflect the values in the home. And I think what we need to do, more than anything, is communicate to the parents in a very kind and pedagogical way, that that is not something that they should want in schools. That what parents should want from schools, what we should all want from schools, is for schools to help young people deliberate about these important issues with people who are different from they are, and hearing views that are different from what they hear at home. Because if we don't do that, we are never going to get beyond what we see right now, which is, unfortunately, people kind of marinating in their own ideological stew."

Hess, D.E. Professor of Curriculum and Instruction, University of Wisconsin-Madison; Senior Vice President, Spencer Foundation. (2014). Deliberation and Bioethics Education: Overview. Presentation to the Bioethics Commission, November 6. Retrieved March 24, 2016 from http://bioethics.gov/node/4321.

To facilitate this reflective process, ethics education should occur in an inclusive environment that encourages open and honest discussion.[183] Teachers must be trained to facilitate these types of discussions, whether or not they teach a dedicated ethics lesson, because conversations among students about differing values are inevitable.

The notion of creating conditions for inclusive discussion should be distinguished from current discourse around creating a safe space, which first emerged to describe an enclave for students trying to avoid racism and sexism. It is now often used to eliminate possible exposure to ideas that might bring emotional discomfort.[184] However, attempting to shield students from ideas or topics that make them uncomfortable can impede the exploratory thinking needed for ethics education and development of deliberative skills needed for democratic citizenship.[185] Rather than excluding these topics from classrooms, teachers should carefully prepare and strategize to introduce these topics in a manner that is tailored for their students' ages, sensitive to diverse cultures and groups, and fair to participants and their views.[186]

The logistics of implementing new programs into existing, often crowded curricula can present a third obstacle.[187] Trying to adhere to national standards such as the Common Core can add to the difficulty.[188] In certain cases, however, ethics discussions, readings, or case studies—particularly cases from bioethics—can fit into current standards and requirements. Moreover, they can enhance the goals that those standards are meant to achieve. For example, the Common Core State Standards emphasize reason-giving—a key skill for democratic deliberation that entails presenting a claim, distinguishing it from opposing claims, and giving reasons and evidence to defend it. This skill manifests in writing requirements for grades 9–12 in which students are expected to construct reasoned arguments by using sufficient evidence. Even students as early as grade 6 develop speaking and listening skills by drawing on facts and details when presenting their claims. Analysis and discussion of an ethical dilemma provides an opportunity for students to become familiar with conceptual and substantial aspects of ethical concerns while fulfilling Common Core skill-building requirements.

Next Generation Science Standards also require that students learn about the nature of science, technology, society, and the environment and the relationships among them.[189] This requirement could be met by considering the ethical and social implications of emerging technologies (e.g., synthetic biology or whole genome sequencing) or developments in neuroscience. Understanding how bioethics topics relate to national curriculum standards in these ways can help teachers and administrators think of ethics and bioethics not as additional subjects that they do not have time to teach, but instead as skill-building topics that can be woven into existing curricula.

A fourth obstacle, most common in the university setting, especially in graduate and postgraduate education, is an incentive structure that discourages faculty from adding ethics to their formal teaching and informal mentoring of students and burgeoning professionals. Cross-disciplinary engagement is often tacitly discouraged simply because such structures as tenure-track hiring and grants incentivize razor-sharp focus on a researcher's chosen topic. Siloed funding can disincentivize incorporation of ethics topics and can act as a barrier to seeking perspectives of other disciplines to help solve ethical dilemmas. Also, programs can be siloed and isolated such that engaging experts from other disciplines (e.g., ethics) is nearly impossible.[190]

As the Bioethics Commission explained in its report, *Gray Matters: Integrative Approaches for Neuroscience, Ethics, and Society*, overcoming these disincentives requires pushing back against them.[191] Universities must secure enough funding and resources to access ethics expertise and convey the importance of and concepts of ethical reasoning to their students and young professionals. If ethics education stops at the undergraduate level, professionals will not have the tools they need to confront ethical challenges specific to their fields. Developing ethics skills in students and faculty requires universities to be supportive of the goals of ethics education throughout a student's lifespan and career development.

Mutual Reinforcement of Deliberation and Ethics Education

Ethics education, through its focus on engagement with values and analytical reasoning, prepares members of communities to engage with and deliberate about morally complex bioethical questions arising in science and technology. In turn, deliberative practices are educational, leading to a more informed and participatory public. These mutually reinforcing functions create a virtuous circle, reflecting the ways in which ethics education and democratic deliberation are linked. Learning to recognize, articulate, and resolve the different ethical challenges we encounter as individuals will foster the skills necessary for deliberating with others about contentious civic concerns we face in our increasingly pluralistic society. In other words, education is crucially important for democratic citizenship.[192] Deliberation can be used as a tool to develop more informed and educated students, professionals, communities, and leaders who can constructively contribute to conversations about morally complex topics—including bioethical ones. The mutual reinforcement of deliberation and ethics education promotes values essential to an engaged and civic-minded population.

> "The expert physicist does not necessarily bring the habits and scruples of the scientist into assessing the policy proposals of candidates for political office. And so we cannot expect that once our students are well-educated in the basic sciences within school they will bring scientific know-how and passion to their deliberation as citizens outside the institution. We need a curriculum for schools in which a substantial part of the curriculum brings established academic disciplines directly to bear on the pressing questions of public policy whose resolution will shape the future of our democracy."
>
> Source: Callan, E., Pigott Family School of Education Professor, Stanford University. (2015, June 4). Comments submitted to the Presidential Commission for the Study of Bioethical Issues, p. 2.

Two of the pedagogical approaches described previously demonstrate the synergy between democratic deliberation and bioethics education. First, the Intercollegiate Ethics Bowl teaches college students how to engage in ethical reasoning by deliberating in teams about specific cases, including bioethics topics. The Ethics Bowl challenges the traditional pedagogical approaches and requires students to engage with the topic and deliberate together, each bringing her own values and ethical reasoning skills to bear. It raises the stakes by using team competition, engaging students in active learning. Second, the high school deliberative classroom activities described by Diana Hess, including town hall meetings, text-based seminars, and discussion groups, teach students topical content and the related ethical issues, as well as skills in articulation and discussion of challenging topics. Activities like these that bring deliberation to life in the classroom demonstrate their value as an educational tool, especially for teaching ethics and bioethics.

Recommendations

Ethics education is important throughout life and can help prepare us for addressing ethical and bioethical issues that arise in everyday life and professional settings. These issues include questions for which no clear right or wrong answer exists, but that require careful consideration and reflection. Such problems include what medical decisions to make—and how best to make them—on behalf of a loved one who is incapacitated, and how to understand the potential social implications of research findings. Many of us also participate as members of private and public associations in our workplace; our local, state, and national governments; and voluntary associations where we encounter broad bioethics topics about which we have concern and over which we might have influence. Education throughout the lifespan that cultivates ethical reasoning and development of moral character can help individuals better meet these challenges in their own lives and in their relationships, and participate in decisions that affect them. Although schools play a key role in developing the values and analytical skills that contribute to an informed population, ethics education is not emphasized in the United States as part of standard curricula. However, great potential exists for incorporation of discussions of ethics into classrooms to develop these skills. Teachers and schools should make use of such educational materials as those developed by the Bioethics Commission and others.

Recommendation 4: Implement Foundational Broad-Based Ethics Education at all Levels

Educators at all levels, from preschool to postsecondary and professional schools, should integrate ethics education across the curriculum to prepare students for engaging with morally complex questions in a diverse range of subjects. Ethics education should include attention to both the development of moral character and virtue as well as the cultivation of ethical reasoning and decision-making skills that can be deployed in a bioethics context. Methods of ethics education should be evidence-based and grounded in best practices.

Development of ethical reasoning skills begins early in childhood, as previously discussed. Questions and case studies with a bioethical component can be an important element of this early education. For example, elementary school students might be asked to think about what questions they would have if they were invited to participate in research. Older elementary school students might be asked to compare theories arrived at by science versus those arrived at by other methods, or to reason through the concept of neurobiologic determinism by answering such discussion questions as, "Are our futures and fates fixed? Does what we do today have any effect on what happens in the future?"[193] Ethics education builds critical thinking and argumentation skills, develops character, and emphasizes the importance of virtue. Those who develop curricula should draw from the empirical evidence about moral development to scaffold questions and topics that are tailored for students' level of thinking at different ages.[194]

Continuing ethics education into secondary school builds on the foundation of character and virtue developed in primary school. In secondary school, students can learn higher order ethical concepts as they relate to their coursework. Programs aimed at training teachers how to introduce bioethics into their classrooms can help ensure teachers have the knowledge and skills to facilitate student engagement.[195] Later, at the university level, as moral development continues to evolve and students begin to specialize, ethics education should also begin to specialize. In undergraduate education, the foundations of character development, decision making, and analytic reasoning skills should be applied to the specific concepts that students are exploring in their coursework.

As programs in ethics education are developed across the lifespan and in diverse settings, creators of these programs should ensure that they are designed in accordance with best evidence and practices. The goals and purposes of each program should be clearly stated, and programs should be evaluated to ensure that they are meeting those goals. Just as schools use evidence amassed over decades about what methods work to teach other topics, so should they design ethics curricula components in accordance with evidence about what works. An effective education in ethical character and reasoning serves everyone well—as current and future patients, caregivers, and community members, all of whom are affected by new developments in science, health, and technology. The importance of ethics education makes evaluating the conditions that lead to successes and failures in building bioethics skills and virtues essential. Such evaluations will then enable building on what is learned to continue improving ethics education.

All individuals should have an opportunity to participate in ethics education to prepare them for the inevitable bioethical decisions they will face. Specific bioethical knowledge and skills should be taught to professionals. In six of its past nine reports, the Bioethics Commission has recommended bioethics training for professionals in fields ranging across medicine, basic science, public health, engineering, and law. This recommendation builds on the Bioethics Commission's past work by urging educators and trainers in these fields to develop continuing bioethics education.

Bioethical challenges within specific professions present questions for which a general ethics education is insufficient. Certain obligations, duties, and virtues are embedded in each profession and social role, and incorporating these into bioethics analyses is important.[196] For example, in its 2013 report, *Anticipate and Communicate: Ethical Management of Incidental and Secondary Findings in the Clinical, Research, and Direct-to-Consumer Contexts*, the Bioethics Commission analyzed the different roles that clinicians, researchers, and direct-to-consumer professionals play in our society and in relation to the patients, participants, and consumers with whom they interact. Thus, rather than making broad recommendations about what any practitioner should do when they discover an incidental finding, the Bioethics Commission made separate recommendations based on the different roles and ethical duties of these professionals in each context.[197]

"I think that the same drive for accountability should animate a Bioethics Commission's thinking and practice with respect to... active participation by citizens. There are...two aspects to this dimension: Public education, the focused effort to lead citizens to an informed understanding of some usually rather complex issue in biomedicine, an effort that might utilize any number of educational methods, and the direct engagement of an informed citizenry in deliberations as a Commission."

Davis, F.D., Director of Bioethics, Geisinger Health System. (2015). Democratic Deliberation in Bioethics. Presentation to the Bioethics Commission, May 27. Retrieved March 25, 2016 from http://bioethics.gov/node/4943.

Additionally, in its 2010 report, *New Directions: The Ethics of Synthetic Biology and Emerging Technologies*, the Bioethics Commission recommended that, because synthetic biology crosses multiple disciplines, bioethics education and training should be developed in relevant fields, including engineering and materials science.[198] Professional ethics seeks to identify and guide professionals' actions on the basis of the moral foundations of their chosen careers, and these actions often need to be explicitly taught. Graduate programs in such professions as nursing and public health ought to help students develop the confidence, reasoning skills, and moral resources they will need to address the distinct ethical considerations of their professional work. Importantly, some graduate programs including laboratory science and public health have independently documented a need to develop critical reasoning skills and moral sensitivity.[199]

Recommendation 5: Develop Bioethics Education and Training for Professionals

Educators at the graduate and professional levels, including in the health care, public health, engineering, and legal fields, should develop, integrate, and emphasize bioethics education to foster continued character development, cultivate a culture of responsibility, and teach the specific skills and bioethical reasoning applicable to the profession.

Administrators and teachers in a wide array of professional fields—including health care, the biosciences, engineering, business, and law—can choose from various options to ensure that their graduates are prepared to recognize and address bioethical issues that arise in their profession. The Bioethics Commission's 2014 report, *Gray Matters: Integrative Approaches for Neuroscience, Ethics, and Society*, described several methods for integrating bioethics into the neuroscience research enterprise. These approaches are not limited to neuroscience, nor necessarily to scientific research. All of the approaches described have an educational component. For example, ethics mentoring programs, collaboration with experts on ethics review boards, and benchside ethics consultation services are some of the ways to incorporate innovative methods for educating professionals who encounter bioethical challenges.[200] Graduate-level training for professionals and students training in those professions—such as master's degree programs in bioethics or health care ethics—can create a cadre of individuals with dual competence in both their field and in ethics. Integrating bioethics into existing professional school curricula also can help develop the necessary skills for ethically competent professionals. These programs could add a bioethics component to each course, have students engage in a separate course that uses a bioethics lens to reflect on a topic, or both. These bioethical elements should be tailored to the specific careers that students are entering and to the kinds of bioethical issues that they are likely to encounter as professionals. For example, in law school, courses that help prepare future attorneys to confront cases involving health care, science, and technology should include a bioethics component for when questions of ethics, not simply law, arise. Competency in bioethics should continue to develop even after graduation—professionals and trainees at all levels can cultivate their ethical competency though formal and informal mentoring programs.

❧

Ethics education at all levels is essential for preparing current and future community members to engage in conversations about challenging and controversial topics. However, introducing ethics and potentially controversial bioethical questions into the classroom can present pedagogical challenges for educators. As described previously, teachers might be concerned that conversations will spiral out of control or that parents, other teachers, or school administrators will object.[201] Teachers in science fields rarely receive training in ethics or in leading discussions and therefore might feel unprepared to implement bioethics curricula.[202] Moreover, many professional incentive structures can discourage incorporating ethics into scientific training.[203]

Educators need support and professional development that prepares them to overcome these obstacles to implementing bioethics education and that rewards them for doing so. Training in ethics and techniques for conducting deliberative discussions in the classroom can help teachers overcome their own and others' hesitancy to engage in bioethics education. Training also can prepare teachers for addressing administrators' and parents' concerns that ethics education seeks to indoctrinate students.

Recommendation 6: Support Opportunities for Teacher Training in Bioethics Education

Education policymakers, teacher training programs, and other funders should support development of teacher training in ethics education to prepare teachers of all subjects to facilitate constructive bioethical conversations in their classrooms. Teacher training programs should anticipate existing educational inequities and provide teachers and students with equitable access to ethics education, with an aim of preparing all students for the bioethical questions that might arise during the course of their lives.

Training programs should prepare educators at all levels to conduct ethics education that provides students with skills and knowledge that will help them navigate through the bioethical decisions they will likely face. Teacher training programs can help direct bioethics education opportunities to be more inclusive. Training programs should be inclusive when considering which teachers are offered training and thus which students are offered ethics education opportunities. They should also consider how to train teachers to think critically about which student contributions to conversation will be perceived as legitimate.[204]

Existing materials for teacher training or professional development programs in bioethics education are a principal resource. Previous training efforts have included workshops, texts that provide instructors with an overview of topics for discussion, teaching manuals, continuing support after initial training, and online resources.[205]

Ethics education, through its focus on analytical reasoning, prepares communities and their members to engage with and deliberate about morally complex bioethical questions in health, science, and technology. In turn, deliberative practices are educational, leading to a more informed and participatory public. These mutually reinforcing functions can create a virtuous circle, reflecting the ways in which ethics education and democratic deliberation are inextricably linked. Deliberation can be used as a tool to develop more informed and educated students, professionals, communities, and leaders. Deliberating about an array of morally complex topics—including bioethical ones—facilitates ethics learning and skill-building. The mutual reinforcement of deliberation and ethics education promotes values essential to an engaged and civic-minded population.

Recommendation 7: Foster Mutual Reinforcement of Deliberation and Ethics Education

Educators and organizers of deliberative activities should use the tools of deliberation and education to facilitate civic engagement about pressing bioethical concerns surrounding developments in health, science, and technology.

Many innovative ways exist to incorporate deliberation into bioethics education. We described several contemporary examples of deliberation enhancing education, including the Ethics Bowl and various deliberative classroom activities. Each of these methods should be implemented with a clear understanding of how they can help achieve educational goals. For example, educators hoping to teach their students about specific substantive topics, while

"[A] team's challenge in preparing for the Ethics Bowl is to identify the key ethical issues raised by each case, and then work out positions on them that everyone on the team agrees are reasonable in the sense that a morally conscientious person could accept the position after careful consideration. And to reach this kind of agreement among themselves each team member has to be able to listen to the others with an open mind. The team members have to be able to consider seriously different views from their own and to appreciate their force, not in the sense of being persuaded necessarily, but in recognizing why a morally responsible person could hold that position or find them persuasive."

Ladenson, R.F., Emeritus Faculty Associate, Center for the Study of Ethics in the Professions, Illinois Institute of Technology. (2015). Ethical and Deliberative Skills across the Lifespan. Presentation to the Bioethics Commission, September 2. Retrieved March 25, 2016 from http://bioethics.gov/node/5267.

honing their civic skills, might choose to incorporate deliberative activities into the classroom. Structured deliberative activities can help revitalize democratic deliberation in our politically polarized society. Deliberative activities are designed to teach "*for* and *with* discussion," meaning that they not only teach a topic through discussion, they are also intended to foster high-quality discussion.[206]

Educators who hope to foster the deliberative skills of mutual understanding and respect for differing positions can adapt the format of the Ethics Bowl in which high school or undergraduate students participate in deliberations on diverse ethics and bioethics topics (e.g., raising the minimum wage or testing an unproven medical intervention on dying patients). Ethics Bowl teams must deliberate, anticipate, and incorporate different perspectives and present a unified response, which can yield educational benefits that a classroom discussion might have difficulty generating.[207] Beyond helping students develop a framework for ethical reasoning and cultivating understanding of a broad range of topics, such activities can foster the critical deliberative skill of taking on the position of an individual with whom they disagree.[208]

Supporting public bioethics education and engaging in deliberation are important functions of bioethics advisory bodies. Bioethics commissions ought to serve as public forums by engaging, educating, listening, and responding to citizens.[209] This Bioethics Commission has actively engaged in and helped to implement deliberative practices and bioethics education. It has made direct contributions to bioethics education by developing teaching tools that are wide-ranging in scope and format and intended to be accessible to both educators and members of the public. These materials draw on research about effective education to ensure that all kinds of learners are able to access the work of the Bioethics Commission, and through that work, engage in some of the most challenging contemporary bioethics topics.

Recommendation 8: Encourage Future Bioethics Commissions to Further Their Deliberative and Educational Roles

Future bioethics commissions should continue to explore, reimagine, and reinvigorate the educational and democratic roles fulfilled and exemplified by such commissions. They also should encourage discourse and civic involvement in developing health, science, and technology policy. The work of bioethics commissions should be used as the foundation for creating educational tools tailored for different levels, from primary school through postgraduate and professional training, that enable teachers to introduce deliberation about contemporary and meaningful bioethics topics in their classrooms.

This Bioethics Commission has demonstrated its commitment to furthering ethics education at all levels by making recommendations calling for both broad public ethics education and specific professional ethics training, as well as developing bioethics educational materials that can be used in a broad range of settings by educators who want to incorporate bioethics into their classrooms. The Bioethics Commission has developed more than 60 educational tools at the time of this printing, and is continuing to develop more, including case studies, deliberation exercises, modules on key bioethics topics, classroom discussion guides, videos, and webinars, all of which are available for free download on the Commission's website. The materials can be used by teachers in high school, college, and graduate school classes; by professionals in the health sciences and technology fields, including clinicians, public health practitioners, and researchers; and by members of the public.

At our 23rd meeting in November 2015, the Bioethics Commission welcomed visitors from Rachel Fink's biology class at Mount Holyoke College in South Hadley, Massachusetts. For more than a decade, she has engaged her students in deliberative activities to help them understand the societal, political, and ethical implications of the science they study in the classroom.[210] At the

November 2015 meeting, students observed Commission members as they engaged in deliberation and solicited comment from experts who came to present their views and recommendations. Students participated by submitting comments to the Commission as the members deliberated. Their participation in this public meeting is an apt illustration of the intersection of bioethics education and public deliberation and is an example of inspiring educational efforts that can build a more informed, engaged, and participatory democracy. Our work in public deliberation and bioethics education has built on the legacy of past bioethics commissions, and we encourage future bioethics commissions to continue in this tradition.

* * *

This discussion about ethics education has wider educational policy implications: the question of *what* subject matter schools should teach often obscures equally important questions about *why* schools should teach. Too often, education policy jumps to *how* questions, focusing on the content of education and assessment methods—what subjects should be taught and mastered and at what age? Although important, these questions are inextricably related to the questions of why students are being educated in the first place. Individuals, families, communities, and societies have different goals for education. Some want the education system to prepare students for an increasingly competitive work environment, whereas others want students to be trained in basic life skills. Others see education as an initial introduction to a lifetime of learning, or they envision education as developing individual talent and potential. Each of these goals is laudable in its own right and ought to underpin conversations about objectives of educational policy reforms. Ethics education, as an integral part of the educational landscape, offers an exploration of these broader goals.

By initiating and encouraging continued conversations about ethics education, the Bioethics Commission hopes to motivate broader reflection on educational policy by setting the question of values and their role in education, front and center. The Bioethics Commission's analysis reveals that educational goals are not mutually exclusive, but often compatible and even complementary. By highlighting bioethics education, the Bioethics Commission's analysis constitutes a call to all those with a stake in teaching and learning to consider the worthwhile goal of fostering thoughtful discussion about our individual and collective values.

This section emphasized the importance of ethics education, from kindergarten through professional development and adult education, for promoting reasoned deliberation about bioethical issues. Moving forward with complex decisions that involve social and ethical dimensions of our lives and that involve deeply held values requires decision makers and the public alike to have a clear understanding of the factors and concerns involved. The only way for us, as a society, to arrive at informed and ethical decisions about important questions concerning advances in science, medicine, and technology is to understand these questions, including their ethical contours. Both education and democratic deliberation are necessary for society to make informed choices about scientific advances.

CONCLUSION

Since its inception, this Bioethics Commission has been committed to the values embedded in democratic deliberation. We hope that this report informs, inspires, and guides future bioethics commissions. We have described our deliberative processes, outlining the key steps in the process of democratic deliberation, and recommended ways of incorporating and extending a deliberative approach to making recommendations and formulating advice on complex ethical challenges in health, science, and technology. As the tenure of this Bioethics Commission draws to a close, we hope that future commissions and advisory bodies at all levels will continue to invoke the values of democratic deliberation as they work to find ways forward on the most pressing bioethical questions that confront our society.

As this report goes to press, the national and international science communities are grappling with the ethical and societal implications of a promising new technology: clustered regularly interspaced short palindromic repeats, or CRISPR.[211] CRISPR is a powerful and efficient technology that is being used by thousands of scientists to edit plant and animal DNA.[212] Researchers hope to use CRISPR to alter human genes to cure and eliminate diseases.[213] Many eminent scientists, ethicists, and members of the public have raised serious concerns about using CRISPR in humans, including potential consequences of an error in genetic engineering, use of the technology for bioterrorism, and unanticipated implications for future generations of altering even such seemingly harmless genes as eye color.[214] Altering a human's germline means altering the genome of all their descendants.[215] Philosophers have previously raised concerns about potential implications of such alterations.[216]

The continued research and use of CRISPR technology is a topic well-suited for democratic deliberation. A host of complex questions concerning how we should use CRISPR technology are open for deliberation. What limits—if any—should we place on its use in humans? Deliberations about this topic should involve diverse stakeholders including scientists and clinicians, as well as ethicists, philosophers, and communities affected by diseases that CRISPR might cure. Deliberating about CRISPR *now* is of utmost importance because the technology is on the cusp of use in humans, including human embryos. A set of deliberative efforts that include stakeholders and members of the public and that foster open discussion and debate is best designed for arriving at actionable decisions about what to do about CRISPR research and use.

The National Academy of Sciences (NAS) has initiated an effort to do just that. NAS is committed to examining both the scientific as well as the "clinical, ethical, legal, and social implications of human genome editing technologies," (e.g., CRISPR).[217] David Baltimore, chair of the NAS committee emphasized, "This is the way decisions get made in a democracy. We may not be representative of all America, but it is a beginning process and an ongoing process. It does establish a precedent for the handling of difficult issues that we can be proud of."[218] NAS held its first international summit in December 2015 and will continue to deliberate, convening experts and members of the public, before releasing a final report by end of 2016 (Figure 5).

FIGURE 5: THE INTERNATIONAL SUMMIT ON HUMAN GENE EDITING

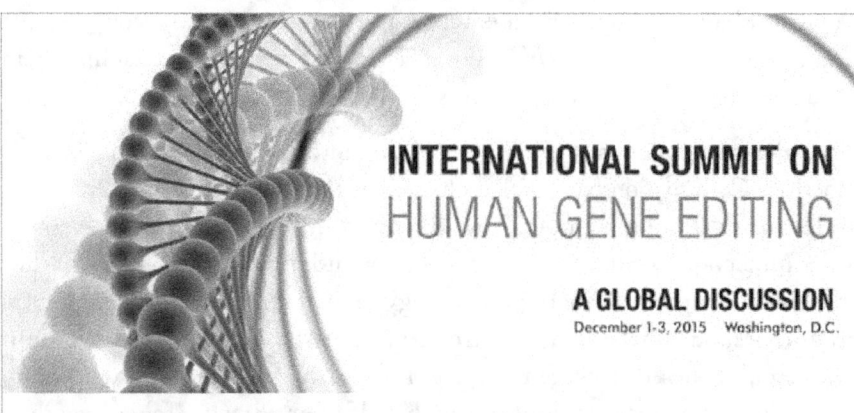

The National Academy of Sciences held an international summit on CRISPR in December of 2015.
Source: http://nationalacademies.org/gene-editing/Gene-Edit-Summit/index.htm.

The deliberative process that NAS is using to guide policy on the emerging CRISPR technology is another excellent example of how policymakers and advisory bodies can and should approach complex problems in health policy and bioethics. The core values of democratic deliberation, including mutual respect and reason-giving, are ideally suited to finding ethical ways forward on pressing matters of common concern, respecting the diverse opinions of stakeholders and arriving at legitimate policy solutions.

* * *

For wise and legitimate decision making about bioethical concerns in a democracy, both experts and the public at large need to understand not only the science, but also attendant values and ethical dimensions. We also must develop skills that enable reasoned ethical argument. Ethics education is necessary for effective deliberation, and deliberation is an excellent tool for ethics education. Teaching communities how to participate in deliberation about real bioethics topics is an efficient and effective way to teach students about the ethical dimensions of health, science, and technology, enabling them to participate in the democratic process.

Bioethics permeates multiple facets of our public and private lives. This Bioethics Commission has tackled challenges that we all face as individuals, professionals, family members, and members of society in an increasingly interconnected world. These questions include, among others, whether and how to employ advancing technology, how researchers and health care providers should behave in certain situations, how governments should handle public health emergencies, and how individuals should incorporate their values when making decisions on behalf of loved ones. Taken together, these questions get to the heart of what it means to be a participant in our democracy and, in an even broader sense, a responsible citizen of the world. Tackling these questions requires careful and reasoned deliberation, as well as a comprehensive understanding of the values that each of us brings to the discussion. Democratic deliberation and ethics education complement one another, elevating the level of discourse about tough bioethical concerns and improving the way our society resolves morally complex challenges in science, technology, and health.

ENDNOTES

1   Gutmann, A. (1999). *Democratic Education*, with a new preface and epilogue. Princeton, NJ: Princeton University Press, pp. xi-xiv, 5-6.

2   Gutmann, A., *supra* note 1, p. 52, et passim.

3   Gutmann, A., and D. Thompson. (2004). *Why Deliberative Democracy?*. Princeton, NJ: Princeton University Press, p. 7.

4   Presidential Commission for the Study of Bioethical Issues (PCSBI). (2010, December). *New Directions: The Ethics of Synthetic Biology and Emerging Technologies*. Washington, DC: PCSBI, p 5.

5   Gutmann, A., and D. Thompson. (1997). Deliberating about bioethics. *Hastings Center Report*, 27(3), 38-41, p. 28.

6   Thompson, D., Alfred North Whitehead Professor of Political Philosophy, Faculty of Arts and Sciences, Professor of Public Policy, John F. Kennedy School of Government, Harvard University (Emeritus). (2015). Facilitating Public Dialogue About Bioethics. Presentation to the Presidential Commission for the Study of Bioethical Issues, September 2. Retrieved March 25, 2016 from http://bioethics.gov/node/5265.

7   Knobloch, K.R., et al. (2014). Empowering citizen deliberation in direct democratic elections: A field study of the 2012 Oregon Citizens' Initiative Review. *Field Actions Science Reports*, 11, 1-10; De Vries, R., et al. (2010). Assessing the quality of democratic deliberation: A case study of public deliberation on the ethics of surrogate consent for research. *Social Science and Medicine*, 70(12), 1896-1903.

8   Primary Ethics. (2015). K-6 Curriculum [Curriculum Framework]. Retrieved March 25, 2016 from http://www.primaryethics.com.au/K-6curriculum.html.

9   Knight, S., Curriculum Author, Primary Ethics Limited, Australia. (2015). Ethical and Deliberative Skills Across the Lifespan. Presentation to the Presidential Commission for the Study of Bioethical Issues, September 2. Retrieved March 25, 2016 from http://bioethics.gov/node/5267.

10 Lee, L.M., Wright, B., and S. Semaan. (2013). Expected ethical competencies of public health professionals and graduate curricula in accredited schools of public health in North America. *American Journal of Public Health*, 103(5), 938-942; Ulrich, C., Associate Professor of Bioethics in Nursing, University of Pennsylvania School of Nursing. (2015). Goals of and Approaches to Bioethics Education. Presentation to the Presidential Commission for the Study of Bioethical Issues, May 27. Retrieved March 25, 2016 from http://bioethics.gov/node/4945.

11 Gutmann, A., *supra* note 1, pp. 282-291, et passim.

12 Dzur, A.W., and D. Levin. (2004). The "nation's conscience:" Assessing bioethics commissions as public forums. *Kennedy Institute of Ethics Journal*, 14(4), 333-360.

13 Dewey, J. (1916). The need of an industrial education in an industrial democracy. In J.A. Boydston (Ed.). (1980). *John Dewey: The Middle Works, 1899-1924*, Vol. 10, p. 139. London, UK: Southern Illinois University Press.

14 Safier, P. (2006). Rationing in Public: The Oregon Health Plan. In A. Gutmann and D. Thompson (Eds.). *Ethics and Politics: Cases and Comments*, Fourth Edition (pp. 332-357). Belmont, CA: Wadsworth.

15 Gutmann, A., *supra* note 1, pp. xi-xiv, 5-6.

16 Gutmann, A., *supra* note 15, p. 52, et passim.

17 Woopen, C., Executive Director, Cologne Center for Ethics, Rights, Economics, and Social Sciences of Health. (2016). Introduction to the 11th Global Summit 2016, Berlin, Global Health – Global Ethics – Global Justice, March 17. Retrieved March 25, 2016 from https://www.globalsummit-berlin2016.de/documents-and-links/GlobalSummitWelcomingSpeechChristianeWoopen.pdf.

18 Gutmann, A., and D. Thompson, *supra* note 3, p. 7.

19 PCSBI, *supra* note 4, p 5.

20 Hess, D.E., and P. McAvoy. (2014). *The Political Classroom: Evidence and Ethics in Democratic Education*. New York, NY: Routledge, p. 5; Parker, W.C. (2003). *Teaching Democracy: Unity and Diversity in Public Life*. New York, NY: Teacher's College Press.

21 Katsnelson, A. (2010, April 14). Freeing human eggs of mutant mitochondria. *Nature*. Retrieved March 22, 2016 from http://www.nature.com/news/2010/100414/full/news.2010.180.html; Sciencewise. (2016). Mitochondria Donation [Webpage]. Retrieved March 22, 2016 from http://www.sciencewise-erc.org.uk/cms/assets/Project-summaries/Mitochondria-donationproject-summary.pdf.

22 United Mitochondrial Disease Foundation (UMDF). (2015). What is Mitochondrial Disease?. Retrieved May 2, 2016 from http://www.umdf.org/site/c.8qKOJ0MvF7LUG/b.7934627/k.3711/What_is_Mitochondrial_Disease.htm; Schaefer, A.M., et al. (2004). The epidemiology of mitochondrial disorders—past, present and future. *Biochimica et Biophysica Acta*, 1659(2-3), 115-120; Elliot, H.R., et al. (2008). Pathogenic mitochondrial DNA mutations are common in the general population. *The American Journal of Human Genetics*, 83(2), 254-260.

23 Human Fertilisation and Embryology Authority (HFEA). (2012, January 19). HFEA to consult on ethics of 'mitochondria transfer' [Press Release]. Retrieved March 22, 2016 from http://www.hfea.gov.uk/6898.html.

24 Ibid.

25 Sciencewise, (2013). Case Study. Mitochondria replacement: A major public dialogue to review the ethical, social and regulatory issues involved in mitochondria replacement and provide the main contribution to HFEA's advice to Government. Retrieved March 22, 2016 from http://www.sciencewise-erc.org.uk/cms/assets/Uploads/SciWiseMitochondria-CS05-04-14.pdf; Watermeyer R., and G. Rowe. (2013, July). Evaluation of the project: "Mitochondria Replacement Consultation." Retrieved March 22, 2016 from http://www.hfea.gov.uk/docs/Mitochondria_evaluation_FINAL_2013.pdf.

26 Human Fertilisation and Embryology Authority (HFEA). (2013, March). Mitochondria Replacement Consultation: Advice to Government, p. 4. Retrieved March 22, 2016 from http://www.hfea.gov.uk/docs/Mitochondria_replacement_consultation_-_advice_for_Government.pdf.

27 Nuffield Council on Bioethics. (2015, 25 February). UK approves regulation on mitochondrial DNA donation [Press Release]. Retrieved March 22, 2016 from http://nuffieldbioethics.org/news/2015/uk-approves-regulation-on-mitochondrial-dna-donation/.

28 Gutmann, A., and D. Thompson, *supra* note 3, pp. 22-23.

29 Gutmann, A., and D. Thompson. (2010). Deliberative Democracy. In R.A. Couto. (Ed.). *Political and Civic Leadership: A Reference Handbook* (pp. 325-332). Washington, DC: Sage Publications, Inc., p. 325; Gutmann, A., and D. Thompson, *supra* note 3, pp. 3, 139; Gutmann, A., and D. Thompson, *supra* note 5, 38-41, p. 38.

30 Gutmann, A. and D. Thompson, *supra* note 3, p. 139; Gutmann, A., and D. Thompson, *supra* note 29.

31 Goold, S.D., et al. (2005). Choosing Healthplans All Together: A deliberative exercise for allocating limited health care resources. *Journal of Health Politics, Policy and Law*, 30(4), 563-601.

32 Danis, M., Ginsburg, M.M., and Goold, S. (2010). Experience in the United States with public deliberation about health insurance benefits using the small group decision exercise, CHAT. *The Journal of Ambulatory Care Management*, 33(3), 205-214.

33 Gutmann, A., and D. Thompson, *supra* note 29.

34 Gutmann, A., and D. Thompson, *supra* note 5, p. 28.

35 Cohen, J. (1997). Deliberation and democratic legitimacy. In Bohman, J. and W. Rehg (Eds.). *Deliberative Democracy: Essays on Reason and Politics* (pp. 67-92). Cambridge, MA: MIT Press, pp. 72-73; Mansbridge, J., et al. (2012). A Systemic Approach to Deliberative Democracy. In J. Parkinson and J. Mansbridge. (Eds.). *Deliberative Systems: Deliberative Democracy at the Large Scale* (pp. 1-26). New York, NY: Cambridge University Press, p. 1.

36 Mansbridge, J. (2007). "Deliberative Democracy" or "Democratic Deliberation"?. In Rosenberg, S.W. (Ed.). *Deliberation, Participation, and Democracy* (pp. 251-271). UK: Palgrave MacMillan, pp. 251-252.

37 Jackson, R., Executive Chair, Sciencewise. (2015). Facilitating public dialogue about bioethics. Presentation to the Presidential Commission for the Study of Bioethical Issues, September 2. Retrieved March 23, 2016 from http://bioethics.gov/node/5265.

38 Gutmann, A., and D. Thompson, *supra* note 5, p. 39.

39 Mill, J.S. (1861). *Considerations on Representative Government*. Kitchener, Canada: Batoche Books, p. 46.

40 Dzur, A.W., and D. Levin, *supra* note 12, p. 341.

41 Gutmann, A., and D. Thompson, *supra* note 5, pp. 40-41; Dzur, A.W., and D. Levin, *supra* note 12, p. 334.

42 Capron, A.M. (2015, May 28). Room for debate. *New York Times*; Capron, A.M., Board Chair, Public Responsibility in Medicine and Research. (2015, May 27). Comments submitted to the Presidential Commission for the Study of Bioethical Issues (PCSBI).

43 Gutmann, A., and D. Thompson, *supra* note 5, p. 40.

44 Mansbridge, J., *supra* note 36.

45 *Federal Advisory Committee Act*. 5 U.S.C. §§ 10, 11.

46 Sarewitz, D. (2015). CRISPR: Science can't solve it. Nature, 522(7557), 413-414.

47 World Wide Views. (2015). World Wide Views on Climate and Energy [Synthesis of Results]. Retrieved March 24, 2016 from http://climateandenergy.wwviews.org/wp-content/uploads/2015/09/WWviews-Result-Report_english_low.pdf.

48 World Wide Views on Climate and Energy. (n.d.) The Method. Retrieved March 24, 2016 from http://climateandenergy.wwviews.org/the-method/.

49 United Nations Framework Convention on Climate Change. (2015, September 25). Global citizens strong support for ambitious Paris agreement: World Wide Views presents consultation results at UN [Press Release]. Retrieved March 24, 2016 from http://newsroom.unfccc.int/unfccc-newsroom/world-wide-views-new-york-press-release/; World Wide Views. (2015, December 16). WWViews: The citizens' voice at COP21 [Blog]. Retrieved March 24, 2016 from http://climateandenergy.wwviews.org/blog/events/wwviews-the-citizens.

50 New York State Department of Health. (n.d.). Task Force on Life and the Law: Reports and Publications [Webpage]. Retrieved March 24, 2016 from http://www.health.ny.gov/regulations/task_force/reports_publications/.

51 New York State Department of Health. (n.d.). Task Force on Life and the Law [Webpage]. Retrieved March 24, 2016 from https://www.health.ny.gov/regulations/task_force/.

52 Ibid.

53 Ibid.

54 American Medical Association. (n.d.). Opinion 9.11 - Ethics Committees in Health Care Institutions. Retrieved March 24, 2016 from http://www.ama-assn.org/ama/pub/physician-resources/medical-ethics/code-medical-ethics/opinion911.page.

55 Ethics in Medicine, University of Washington School of Medicine. (n.d.). Ethics Committees, Programs and Consultations. Retrieved March 24, 2016 from https://depts.washington.edu/bioethx/topics/ethics.html.

56 American Medical Association, *supra* note 54; McGee, G., et al. (2002). Successes and failures of hospital ethics committees: A national survey of ethics committee chairs. *Cambridge Quarterly of Healthcare Ethics*, 11(1), 87-93; McGee, G., et al. (2001). A national study of ethics committees. *The American Journal of Bioethics*, 1(4), 60-64.

57 Presidential Commission for the Study of Bioethical Issues (PCSBI). (2013, March). *Safeguarding Children: Pediatric Medical Countermeasure Research*. Washington, DC: PCSBI, pp. vii-viii, 4-5.

58 King, J. C., et al. (2015). Evaluation of anthrax vaccine safety in 18 to 20 year olds: A first step towards age de-escalation studies in adolescents. *Vaccine*, 33(21), 2470-2476.

59 Presidential Commission for the Study of Bioethical Issues (PCSBI). (2015, March). *Gray Matters: Topics at the Intersection of Neuroscience, Ethics, and Society*. Washington, DC: PCSBI.

60 Kim, S.Y.H., et al. (2009). Assessing the public's views in research ethics controversies: Deliberative democracy and bioethics as natural allies. *Journal of Empirical Research on Human Research Ethics*, 4(4), 3-16; Kim, S.Y.H., et al. (2011). Effect of public deliberation on attitudes toward surrogate consent for dementia research. *Neurology*, 77(24), 2097-2104.

61 Proposal to Improve Rules Protecting Human Research Subjects, 80 Fed. Reg. 173, 53969 (September 8, 2015).

62 Mansbridge, J., *supra* note 36.

63 Gutmann, A., and D. Thompson, *supra* note 5, 38-41.

64 Community Ethics Committee. (2014, February). Organ Transplant Recipient Listing Criteria. Retrieved March 24, 2016 from http://bioethics.hms.harvard.edu/sites/g/files/mcu336/f/CEC-REPORT-Organ-Transplant-Listing-Criteria-February-2014.pdf.

65 Willard, J. (2015). Structuring bioethics education: The question, the disciplines, and the integrative challenge. *Ethics and Social Welfare*, 9(3), 280-296.

66 Community Ethics Committee. (2015, July 4). Comments submitted to the Presidential Commission for the Study of Bioethical Issues (PCSBI), p. 1.

67 Gutmann, A. (2011). The ethics of synthetic biology: Guiding principles for emerging technologies. *Hastings Center Report*, 41(4), 17-22, p. 20.

68 PCSBI, *supra* note 57.

69 Presidential Commission for the Study of Bioethical Issues. (PCSBI). (2015, February). *Ethics and Ebola: Public Health Planning and Response*. Washington, DC: PCSBI, p. 8.

70 UNICEF. (2015, January). Liberia: Ebola Situation Report no. 69. Retrieved March 25, 2015 from http://www.unicef.org/appeals/files/UNICEF_Liberia_SitRep_14_January_2015.pdf.

71 Pitts, D. (2015). Guinea: Meaningful Messengers [Presentation Abstract, 2015 National Conference on Health Communication, Marketing, & Media]. Retrieved March 25, 2016 from https://cdc.confex.com/cdc/nphic15/webprogram/Paper36118.html.

72 Fishkin, J.S., and R.C. Luskin. (2005). Experimenting with a democratic ideal: Deliberative polling and public opinion. *Acta Politica*, 40(3), 284-298.

73 PCSBI, *supra* note 59.

74 PCSBI, *supra* note 69, pp. 8-9.

75 Fishkin, J.S. (2006, March 1). The nation in a room: Turning public opinion into policy. *Boston Review*. Retrieved March 25, 2016 from https://www.bostonreview.net/james-fishkin-nation-in-a-room-turning-public-opinion-into-policy.

76 Ibid.

77 Ibid; Gastil, J., Head and Professor, Communication Arts and Sciences and Political Science, The Pennsylvania State University. (2015). Fostering and measuring success in ethics and deliberation. Presentation to the Presidential Commission for the Study of Bioethical Issues, September 2. Retrieved March 25, 2016 from http://bioethics.gov/node/5268.

78 Gastil, J., *supra* note 77.

79 Mansbridge, J., *supra* note 36, p. 11.

80 Gutmann, A., and D. Thompson, *supra* note 5, pp. 3-4.

81 Fishkin, J.S., et al. (2010). Deliberative democracy in an unlikely place: Deliberative polling in China. *British Journal of Political Science*, 40(2), 435-448; Danis, M., Head, Section on Ethics and Health Policy, Department of Bioethics, National Institutes of Health (NIH) Clinical Center. (2015). Facilitating public dialogue about bioethics. Presentation to the Presidential Commission for the Study of Bioethical Issues, September 2. Retrieved March 25, 2016 from http://bioethics.gov/node/5265.

[82] Luskin, R. C., et al. (2014). Deliberating across deep divides. *Political Studies*, 62(1), 116-135; Evans, F., Deliberative Poll Participant, What's Next California. (2015). Facilitating public dialogue about bioethics. Presentation to the Presidential Commission for the Study of Bioethical Issues, September 2. Retrieved March 25, 2016 from http://bioethics.gov/node/5265.

[83] Sciencewise. (n.d.). Background. Retrieved March 25, 2016 from http://www.sciencewise-erc.org.uk/cms/background/.

[84] Sciencewise, *supra* note 25.

[85] Jackson, R., *supra* note 37.

[86] Gastil, J., Richards, R.C., and K.R. Knobloch, (2014). Vicarious deliberation: How the Oregon Citizens' Initiative Review influenced deliberation in mass elections. *International Journal of Communication*, 8, 62-89.

[87] Knobloch, K.R., et al., *supra* note 7.

[88] Safier, P., *supra* note 14.

[89] Ibid.

[90] Ibid.

[91] Ibid.

[92] Ibid.

[93] S. 27, 65th Legis. Assemb., § 4 (Or. 1989).

[94] Safier, P., *supra* note 14.

[95] Ibid; Fleck, L.M. (1994). Just caring: Oregon, health care rationing, and informed democratic deliberation. *Journal of Medicine and Philosophy*, 19(4), 367-388.

[96] S. 27, *supra* note 93.

[97] Safier, P., *supra* note 14; Fleck, L.M., *supra* note 95.

[98] Safier, P., *supra* note 14, p. 337.

[99] Thompson, D., *supra* note 6.

[100] PCSBI, *supra* note 69.

[101] Kim, S.Y.H., et al, *supra* note 60.

[102] Knobloch, K.R., et al., *supra* note 7; De Vries, R., et al., *supra* note 7.

[103] Thompson, D.F. (2008). Deliberative Democratic Theory and Empirical Political Science. *American Review of Political Science*, 11, 497-520.

[104] King, Jr., M.L. (1947). The Purpose of Education. In Carson et al (Eds.). (1992). *The Papers of Martin Luther King, Jr., Volume I: Called to Serve, January 1929-June 1951* (pp. 123-124). Berkeley, CA: University of California Press, p. 124.

[105] Presidential Commission for the Study of Bioethical Issues (PCSBI). (2011, September). *"Ethically Impossible" STD Research in Guatemala from 1946 to 1948*. Washington, DC: PCSBI, p. 2-3.

[106] Ibid; Jones, J.H. (1993). *Bad Blood: The Tuskegee Syphilis Experiment*. New York, NY: The Free Press.

[107] U.S. Department of Education (ED). (n.d.). Every Student Succeeds Act (ESSA). Retrieved March 25, 2016 from http://www.ed.gov/essa.

[108] Commission on the Teaching of Bioethics. (1976). Part Two: The Scope of Bioethics Teaching. In *The Teaching of Bioethics* (pp. 14-60). Hastings-on-Hudson, NY: The Hastings Center: Institute of Society, Ethics, and the Life Sciences, p. 49.

[109] Lee L.M., and F.A. McCarty. (2016). Emergence of a discipline? Growth in U.S. postsecondary bioethics degrees. *Hastings Center Report*, 46(2), 19-21.

[110] Commission on the Teaching of Bioethics, *supra* note 108; Andre, J. (2002). *Bioethics as Practice*. Chapel Hill, North Carolina: University of North Carolina Press; Sugarman, J., and Sulmasy, D. P. (2010). Part I: Overview. In Sugarman, J., and Sulmasy, D. P. (Eds.). *Methods in Medical Ethics*. Second Edition. Washington, DC: Georgetown University Press, pp. 3-36.

[111] Commission on the Teaching of Bioethics, *supra* note 108, p. 17.

[112] Franklin, B. (1976) [1749]. Proposals Relating to the Education of Youth in Pennsylvania. In *Journal of General Education*, 28(3), 256-261.

[113] Miller, G. (2008). Students learn how, not what, to think about difficult issues. *Science*, 322(5899), 186-187.

[114] Joffe, S., Emanuel and Robert Hart Associate Professor of Medical Ethics and Health Policy, University of Pennsylvania Perelman School of Medicine. (2015). Goals of and Approaches to Bioethics Education. Presentation to the Presidential Commission for the Study of Bioethical Issues, May 27. Retrieved March 23, 2016 from http://bioethics.gov/node/4945.

[115] Gutmann, A., *supra* note 1, pp. 232-255.

[116] Mill, J.S. (1867). Inaugural address at the University of St. Andrews. In J.M. Robson (Eds). (1984). *Collected Works, Volume XXI: Essays on Equality, Law, and Education* (pp. 215-257). Toronto, Canada: University of Toronto Press, p. 217.

[117] Ibid, p. 218.

[118] Smetana, J.G. (1981). Preschool children's conceptions of moral and social rules. *Child Development*, 52(4), 1333-1336.

[119] Primary Ethics. (n.d.). Our History. Retrieved March 23, 2016 from http://www.primaryethics.com.au/ourhistory.html.

[120] Primary Ethics. (n.d.). K-6 Curriculum. Retrieved March 23, 2016 from http://www.primaryethics.com.au/K-6curriculum.html.

[121] Knight, S., *supra* note 9.

[122] Character.org, (n.d.). Vision and Mission [Webpage]. Retrieved March 23, 2016 from http://character.org/about/vision-and-mission/.

[123] Character.org, (n.d.). Character.org Announces Record Number of Applicants with its Schools of Character Application. Retrieved March 23, 2016 from http://character.org/articles/character-org-announces-record-number-of-applicants-with-its-schools-of-character-application/.

[124] Bishop, L.J., and L. Szobota. (2015). Teaching bioethics at the secondary school level. *Hastings Center Report*, 45(5), 19-25; Others have documented how learning through discussion (regardless of content) occurs more frequently in courses for high-achieving students. See, Nystrand, M., et al. (2003). Questions in time: Investigating the structure and dynamics of unfolding classroom discourse. *Discourse Processes*, 35(2), 135–198.

[125] Schmidt, W.H., et al. (2015). The role of schooling in perpetuating educational inequality: An international perspective. *Educational Researcher*, 44(7), 371-386.

[126] Dávila, A. and M.T. Mora. (2007). An assessment of civic engagement and educational attainment. Retrieved March 23, 2016 from http://www.civicyouth.org/PopUps/FactSheets/FS_Mora.Davila.pdf.

[127] Bishop, L.J., and L. Szobota., *supra* note 124.

[128] Jennings, B., et al. (1990). *New Choices, New Responsibilities: Ethical Issues in the Life Sciences*. Briarcliff Manor, NY: The Hastings Center.

[129] Lundmark, C. (2002). Improving the science curriculum with bioethics. *BioScience*, 52(10), 881.

[130] Bishop, L.J., and L. Szobota., *supra* note 124.

[131] National Institutes of Health (NIH) Clinical Center Department of Bioethics. (2009). Exploring Bioethics [Curriculum Supplement]. Retrieved March 25, 2016 from https://science.education.nih.gov/supplements/nih9/bioethics/guide/pdf/teachers_guide.pdf.

[132] Kennedy Institute of Ethics. (n.d.) High School Bioethics Curriculum Project: Workshop Archive. Retrieved March 23, 2016 from https://highschoolbioethics.georgetown.edu/archive/workshops/; Lundmark, C., *supra* note 129; NIH, *supra* note 131.

[133] Hess, D. (2009). *Controversy in the Classroom.* New York, NY: Routledge, p. 57.

[134] Ibid, pp. 56-60.

[135] Ibid, p. 61.

[136] Ibid, pp. 60-65.

[137] Ibid, p. 67.

[138] Ibid, pp. 65-71.

[139] Ibid, p. 76.

[140] Little, M., Director, Kennedy Institute of Ethics; Professor of Philosophy, Georgetown University. (2015). Goals of and Approaches to Bioethics Education. Presentation to the Presidential Commission for the Study of Bioethical Issues, May 27. Retrieved March 23, 2016 from http://bioethics.gov/node/4945.

[141] Ibid.

[142] Ibid.

[143] Callahan, D. (1980). Goals in the Teaching of Ethics. In D. Callahan and S. Bok (Eds.). *Ethics Teaching in Higher Education* (pp. 61-80). New York, NY: Plenum Press, pp. 79-80.

[144] Ibid.

[145] Ladenson, R. (2001). The educational significance of the ethics bowl. *Teaching Ethics*, 1(1), 63-78, 68.

[146] Ibid.

[147] For a list of all past national and regional IEB cases, see Association for Practical and Professional Ethics. (n.d.). Cases, Rules, and Guidelines. Retrieved March 24, 2016 from http://appe.indiana.edu/ethics-bowl/previous-cases/.

[148] Skipper, R.B. et al., (2016). Cases for the Twentieth Intercollegiate Ethics Bowl National Championship [Case Packet]. Retrieved March 29, 2016 from http://appe.indiana.edu/files/9014/5288/0828/National_Ethics_Bowl_Cases_2016_corrected.pdf.

[149] Arora, K. et al. (2016). 2016 Bioethics Bowl Case Packet [Case Packet]. Retrieved March 29, 2016 from http://nubc2016.com/wp-content/uploads/2014/12/2016-Bioethics-Bowl-Case-Packet.pdf; National Undergraduate Bioethics Conference 2014. (n.d.). Bioethics Bowl Competition. Retrieved from https://nubc2014.wordpress.com/13-2/.

[150] Association for Practical and Professional Ethics (APPE). (n.d.). About Ethics Bowl: Intercollegiate Ethics Bowl. Retrieved March 22, 2016 from http://appe.indiana.edu/ethics-bowl/ethics-bowl/.

[151] Illinois Institute of Technology Center for the Study of Ethics in the Professions. (n.d.). QED: The Ethical Debaters. Retrieved 3/22/2016 from http://ethics.iit.edu/teaching/ethics-bowl/iit-team.

[152] Solomon, M., President, The Hastings Center; Clinical Professor of Anaesthesia, Harvard Medical School. (2013). Integrating Ethics and Neuroscience through Education. Presentation to the Presidential Commission for the Study of Bioethical Issues, December 18. Retrieved March 24, 2016 from http://bioethics.gov/node/3238.

[153] Pellegrino, E.D. and T.R. McElhinney. (1982). Teaching Ethics, the Humanities, and Human Values in Medical Schools: A Ten-Year Overview. Washington, D.C.: Institute on Human Values in Medicine, Society for Health and Human Values.

[154] Lehmann, L.S., et al. (2004). A survey of medical ethics education at U.S. and Canadian medical schools. *Academic Medicine*, 79(7), 682-689.

[155] Ibid; Macklin, R. (1993). Teaching bioethics to future health professionals: A case-based clinical model. *Bioethics*, 7(2-3), 200-206; Carrese, J.A., et al. (2015). The essential role of medical ethics education in achieving professionalism: The Romanell report. *Academic Medicine*, 90(6), 744-752.

[156] Lee, L.M., Wright, B., and S. Semaan, *supra* note 10.

[157] Ulrich, C., *supra* note 10; Grady, C., et al. (2008). Does ethics education influence the moral action of practicing nurses and social workers? *American Journal of Bioethics*, 8(4), 4-11.

[158] Solomon, M., *supra* note 152; Anderson, M.A. (2016). Pedagogical support for responsible conduct of research training. *Hastings Center Report*, 46(1), 18-25.

[159] Solomon, M., *supra* note 152.

[160] Anderson, M.A., *supra* note 158; Presidential Commission for the Study of Bioethical Issues (PCSBI). (2014, May). *Gray Matters: Integrative Approaches for Neuroscience, Ethics, and Society*. Washington, DC: PCSBI.

[161] Sulmasy, D.P. (2000). Should medical schools be schools for virtue? *Journal of General Internal Medicine*, 15(7), 514-516.

[162] Anderson, M.S., et al. (2007). What do mentoring and training in the responsible conduct of research have to do with scientists' misbehavior? Findings from a national survey of NIH-funded scientists. *Academic Medicine*, 82(9), 853-860.

[163] Wald, H.S., et al. (2015). Professional identify formation in medical education for humanistic, resilient physicians: Pedagogic strategies for bridging theory to practice. *Academic Medicine*, 90(6), 753-760.

[164] Sabatino, C.P. (2014). Advance care planning tools that educate, engage, and empower. *Public Policy & Aging Report*, 24(3), 107-111; Tucker, E. (2014, March 22). What on earth is a death cafe? *The Guardian*. Retrieved March 24, 2016 from http://www.theguardian.com/lifeandstyle/2014/mar/22/death-cafe-talk-about-dying; Health Ethics Australia. (n.d.) Building health ethics literacy for Australians [Webpage]. Retrieved March 24, 2016 from http://www.healthethicsaustralia.com/our-activities.

[165] Alzheimer's Association. (2011). Protection of Participants in Research Studies. Retrieved March 24, 2016 from http://www.alz.org/documents_custom/statements/Protection_of_Participants_in_Research.pdf.

[166] Alzheimer's Association. (2012). Ethical Issues and Dementia. Retrieved March 24, 2016 from https://www.alz.org/library/downloads/ethics_rl2012.doc.pdf.

[167] AARP. (2000). AARP Survey on Lifelong Learning [Research Report]. Retrieved March 24, 2016 from http://assets.aarp.org/rgcenter/general/lifelong.pdf, pp. 15-16.

[168] Ibid, pp. 16.

[169] Ibid, pp. 37, 78.

[170] PCSBI, *supra* note 160, pp. 12-18.

[171] Bishop, L.J., and L. Szobota., *supra* note 124; Chowning, J.T. (2005). How to have a successful science and ethics discussion. *Science Teacher*, 72(9), 46-50; Chowning, J.T. (2009). Why societal issues belong in science class. *Science Teacher*, 76(7), 8; The Wellcome Trust. (2001). Valuable Lessons: Engaging with the social context of science in schools [Recommendations and summary of research findings]. Retrieved March 24, 2016 from http://www.wellcome.ac.uk/stellent/groups/corporatesite/@msh_peda/documents/web_document/wtd003446.pdf.

[172] Hess, D.E., and P. McAvoy, *supra* note 20, p. 6.

[173] Bishop, L.J., and L. Szobota., *supra* note 124, p. 21.

[174] Northwest Association for Biomedical Research. (n.d.). Teacher Center [Webpage]. Retrieved March 24, 2016 from https://www.nwabr.org/teacher-center; Chowning, J.T. and P. Fraser. (2007). An Ethics Primer [Instructor guide]. Retrieved March 24, 2016 from https://www.nwabr.org/sites/default/files/NWABR_EthicsPrimer7.13.pdf.

175 Miller, G., *supra* note 113.

176 NIH, *supra* note 131.

177 Carrese, J.A., et al., *supra* note 155.

178 DuBois, J.M., and J. Burkemper. (2002). Ethics education in U.S. medical schools: A study of syllabi. *Academic Medicine*, 77(5), 432-437.

179 Ripple, C., Associate Director for Education Research and Engagement, Duke University Social Science Research Institute. (2015). Fostering and Measuring Success in Ethics and Deliberation. Presentation to the Presidential Commission for the Study of Bioethical Issues, September 2. Retrieved March 24, 2016 from http://bioethics.gov/node/5268.

180 Ibid.

181 Hess, D.E., and P. McAvoy, *supra* note 20, p. 6; McAvoy, P., and D. Hess. (2013). Classroom deliberation in an era of political polarization. *Curriculum Inquiry*, 43(1), 14-47, p. 21; Chowning, J.T. (2005), *supra* note 171; Miller, G., *supra* note 113.

182 Bishop, L., Head of Academic Programs, Kennedy Institute of Ethics, Georgetown University. (2015). Implementing Innovations in Ethics Education. Presentation to the Presidential Commission for the Study of Bioethical Issues, November 17. Retrieved March 23, 2016 from http://bioethics.gov/node/5358.

183 Commission on the Teaching of Bioethics, *supra* note 108, p. 16.

184 Sherlock, R. (2015, November 28). How political correctness rules in America's student 'safe spaces.' *The Telegraph*. Retrieved March 24, 2016 from http://www.telegraph.co.uk/news/worldnews/northamerica/usa/12022041/How-political-correctness-rules-in-Americas-student-safe-spaces.html; Lukianoff, G., and J. Haidt. (2015, September). The coddling of the American mind. *The Atlantic*. Retrieved on March 24, 2016 from http://www.theatlantic.com/magazine/archive/2015/09/the-coddling-of-the-american-mind/399356/.

185 Steiner, D.M. (2014, February 21). The new common core assessments: How they could stop patronizing our students. *Huffington Post*. Retrieved March 24, 2016 from http://www.huffingtonpost.com/david-m-steiner/the-new-common-core-asses_b_4809973.html.

186 Hess, D.E., and P. McAvoy, *supra* note 20, p. 6.

187 Chowning, J.T., *supra* note 171.

188 Common Core State Standards Initiative. (2010). Common Core State Standards for English Language Arts & Literacy in History/Social Studies, Science, and Technical Subjects [Educational Standards]. Retrieved March 25, 2016 from http://www.corestandards.org/wp-content/uploads/ELA_Standards1.pdf, pp. 45, 49-50.

189 Next Generation Science Standards. (2013). APPENDIX J–Science, Technology, Society and the Environment. Retrieved March 13, 2016 from http://nextgenscience.org/sites/default/files/APPENDIX%20J_0.pdf.

190 PCSBI, *supra* note 160, p. 24.

191 PCSBI, *supra* note 160, pp. 24-30.

192 Gutmann, A., *supra* note 1, pp. 282-291, et passim.

193 Primary Ethics, *supra* note 8.

194 Knight, S., *supra* note 9.

195 Miller, G., *supra* note 113.

196 Pellegrino, E.D. (2001). The internal morality of clinical medicine: a paradigm for the ethics of the helping and healing professions. *Journal of Medicine and Philosophy*, 26(6), 559-579; Andre, J. (1991). Role morality as a complex instance of ordinary morality. *American Philosophical Quarterly*, 28(1), 73-80.

197 Presidential Commission for the Study of Bioethical Issues (PCSBI). (2013, December). *Anticipate and Communicate: Ethical Management of Incidental and Secondary Findings in the Clinical, Research, and Direct-to-Consumer Contexts*. Washington, DC: PCSBI.

[198] PCSBI, *supra* note 4, p. 11.

[199] Lee, L.M., Wright, B., and S. Semaan, *supra* note 10; Ulrich, C., *supra* note 10.

[200] PCSBI, *supra* note 160, pp. 12-23.

[201] Hess, D.E., and P. McAvoy, *supra* note 20, p. 6; Chowning, J.T., *supra* note 171; Miller, G., *supra* note 113.

[202] Chowning, J.T., et al. (2012). Fostering critical thinking, reasoning, and argumentation skills through bioethics education. *PloS one*, 7(5), e36791; NIH, *supra* note 131.

[203] PCSBI, *supra* note 160, p. 24.

[204] McAvoy, P., and D. Hess., *supra* note 181, pp. 24-25.

[205] Bishop, L.J., and L. Szobota., *supra* note 124.

[206] Hess, D., *supra* note 133, p. 76. [Original emphasis].

[207] Ladenson, R., *supra* note 145, pp. 68-79.

[208] Ibid, p. 68.

[209] Dzur, A.W., and D. Levin, *supra* note 12, 333-360.

[210] Fink, R.D. (2002). Cloning, stem cells, and the current national debate: Incorporating ethics into a large introductory biology course. *Cell Biology Education*, 1(4), 132-144.

[211] Cong, L., et al. (2013). Multiplex genome engineering using CRISPR/Cas systems. *Science*, 339(6121), 819-823; Jinek, M., et al. (2012). A programmable dual-RNA–guided DNA endonuclease in adaptive bacterial immunity. *Science*, 337(6096), 816-821; Knoepfler, P. (2015, November 30). We need a moratorium on genetically modifying humans. *Slate*. Retrieved March 25, 2016 from http://www.slate.com/articles/health_and_science/science/2015/11/crispr_genetic_modification_should_not_be_used_on_humans.html.

[212] Knoepfler, P., *supra* note 211.

[213] Ledford, H. (2015). CRISPR, the disruptor. *Nature*, 522(7554), 20-24; Gene editing tool can remove HIV DNA from infected cells. (2016, March 27). *News Independent*. Retrieved March 30, 2016 from http://www.thenewsindependent.com/gene-editing-tool-can-remove-hiv-dna-infected-cells/11229/.

[214] Ledford, H., *supra* note 213; Krieger, L.M. (2015, December 3). Gene editing: Don't use in human reproduction, says panel. *Santa Cruz Sentinel*. Retrieved March 25, 2016 from http://www.santacruzsentinel.com/article/ZZ/20151203/NEWS/151208848; Basulto, D. (2015, November 4). Everything you need to know about why CRISPR is such a hot technology. *Washington Post*. Retrieved March 25, 2016 from https://www.washingtonpost.com/news/innovations/wp/2015/11/04/everything-you-need-to-know-about-why-crispr-is-such-a-hot-technology/.

[215] Basulto, D., *supra* note 214.

[216] Sandel, M.J. (2004, April). The case against perfection. *Atlantic Monthly*. Retrieved March 25, 2016 from http://www.theatlantic.com/magazine/archive/2004/04/the-case-against-perfection/302927/; Habermas, J. (2003). *The Future of Human Nature*. Cambridge, UK: Polity Press.

[217] The National Academies of Sciences, Engineering, Medicine. (n.d.) About the Study. Retrieved March 25, 2016 from http://nationalacademies.org/gene-editing/consensus-study/about/index.htm.

[218] Krieger, L.M., *supra* note 214.

APPENDICES

Appendix I: Steps for Deliberation

This appendix provides a condensed guide for how to conduct democratic deliberation in any context. Facilitators of deliberative processes can use this guide as a resource to determine whether deliberation is appropriate for the question at hand, and as a guide to the steps for conducting the process.[1]

 Step I. Begin with an open policy question

- Choose an open question and consider distinct points of view. The question should have an applied component, including questions about how to move forward and what should be done.
- *Example in bioethics*: The Bioethics Commission deliberated about numerous open questions, including: What are the ethical implications of the emerging science of synthetic biology and how should we address them? Should the government move ahead with pediatric testing of medical countermeasures in the face of unknown or unknowable risk of a bioterrorism event? What are the core ethical standards that should guide neuroscience research and its applications.

 Step II. Time deliberation for maximum impact

- Allow ample lead time for deliberation before a decision becomes absolutely necessary. In the case of an ongoing emergency situation, conduct deliberation simultaneously, and apply results as soon as possible.
- *Example in bioethics*: In the Bioethics Commission's work on Ethics and Ebola, an ongoing public health emergency, deliberations were conducted quickly with the hope of providing policy guidance in the midst of an emergency. In its work on pediatric medical countermeasures the Bioethics Commission's deliberations were conducted in advance of a potential bioterrorism attack, so that guidance could be provided with ample time to implement ethical policy and sound science.

 Step III. Invite input from experts and the public

- Use sound and relevant information to inform the deliberation. If new information emerges, integrate it into the deliberation. Evaluate evidence through an established and reliable mechanism before and during deliberation. Make established facts, in the form of accessible background materials, available to all participants.

---

[1] For a more in-depth discussion of this process, including resources for further reading, see Chapter 2 of this report.

Step III continued

- *Example in bioethics*: For each of its topics, the Bioethics Commission sought to uncover all relevant facts and emerging evidence through thorough background research, input from members of the public, and testimony from invited experts and community members, including individuals from affected communities.

 ## Step IV. Foster open discussion and debate

- Cultivate an environment that encourages participants in the deliberation to practice mutual respect and reason-giving.

- *Example in bioethics*: After hearing testimony from experts and community members at each meeting, the Bioethics Commission engaged in roundtable discussions with speakers to allow for an exchange of ideas and perspectives. The background and experiences of the experts and community members, combined with that of the Bioethics Commission members fostered thoughtful and robust discussion, enhanced by the integration of public comment.

 ## Step V. Develop detailed, actionable recommendations

- Feed decisions back into the policymaking process whenever possible, either by making the results of deliberation binding, or by asking participants to develop a set of recommendations that policymakers can use to guide their decisions.

- *Example in bioethics*: In all of its reports, the Bioethics Commission developed detailed, actionable recommendations, many of which have been implemented into policy, law, or practice. For example, in its report *Privacy and Progress in Whole Genome Sequencing*, the Bioethics Commission recommended that laws be drafted to protect individuals' genetic privacy. The California legislature introduced such a law, modeled after the Bioethics Commission's recommendation.[1] In the Bioethics Commission's report *Anticipate and Communicate: Ethical Management of Incidental and Secondary Findings in the Clinical, Research, and Direct-to-Consumer Contexts*, it recommended that clinicians respect a patient's preference to opt-out of receiving incidental and secondary findings, consistent with the clinician's fiduciary duty. The American College of Medical Genetics and Genomics (ACMG) initially concluded that these findings be reported without consideration of patient preferences, but subsequent to the Bioethics Commission's recommendation, the ACMG updated its stance, allowing patients to opt out of receiving such findings if desired.

[1] See more at: http://blog.bioethics.gov/2013/03/12/privacy-and-progress-inspires-california-genetic-information-privacy-bill/.

Appendix II: List of the Bioethics Commission's Educational Materials by Format*

Case Studies

Public Health Case Studies Introduction
Communicating During a Public Health Emergency
Ethical Use of Liberty-restricting Public Health Measures

Conversation Series

For Consumers: A Guide to Incidental Findings
For Patients: A Guide to Incidental Findings
For Research Participants: A Guide to Incidental Findings

Deliberative Scenarios

Guide to Classroom Deliberation for Students and Teachers
Deliberative Scenario: The Use of Prescription Stimulants for Enhanced
    Academic Performance
Teacher Companion for *Deliberative Scenario: The Use of Prescription Stimulants for
    Enhanced Academic Performance*
Deliberative Scenario: Law Enforcement Access to a University's Genetic Database
Teacher Companion for *Deliberative Scenario: Law Enforcement Access to a
    University's Genetic Database*

Discussion Guides

Classroom Discussion Guide on Ethics and Neuroscience
Classroom Discussion Guide on Ethics and Public Health Emergencies

Empirical Research Resources

Guatemala Subject Data Spreadsheet
Human Subjects Research Landscape Project – Analysis Dataset

Primers

For Clinicians: Incidental and Secondary Findings
For Direct-to-Consumer Providers: Incidental and Secondary Findings
For IRB Members: Incidental and Secondary Findings
For Researchers: Incidental and Secondary Findings
For Researchers: Neuroscience and Consent Capacity

Videos

Promoting and Providing Materials for Bioethics Education
The Role of a Presidential Bioethics Commission
Who is the Bioethics Commission?
Challenging Topics for the Bioethics Commission
Incidental Findings: Why Practitioners Need a Plan
Gray Matters
What Goes into Successful Deliberation?

Study Guides

Study Guide to *"Ethically Impossible" STD Research in Guatemala from 1946 to 1948*
Study Guide to *"Ethically Impossible" STD Research in Guatemala from 1946 to 1948*
(Spanish translation)

Topic-Based Modules (listed by topic)

COMMUNITY ENGAGEMENT
  Community Engagement Background
  Community Engagement in *New Directions: The Ethics of Synthetic Biology and Emerging Technologies*
  Community Engagement in *Moral Science: Protecting Participants in Human Subjects Research*
  Community Engagement in *Privacy and Progress in Whole Genome Sequencing*

COMPENSATION
  Compensation Background
  Compensation in *Moral Science: Protecting Participants in Human Subjects Research*
  Compensation in Safeguarding *Children: Pediatric Medical Countermeasure Research*

INFORMED CONSENT
  Informed Consent Background
  Informed Consent in *"Ethically Impossible" STD Research in Guatemala from 1946 to 1948*
  Informed Consent in *Privacy and Progress in Whole Genome Sequencing*
  Informed Consent in *Safeguarding Children: Pediatric Medical Countermeasure Research*
  Informed Consent in *Anticipate and Communicate: Ethical Management of Incidental and Secondary Findings in the Clinical, Research, and Direct-to-Consumer Contexts*
  Informed Consent in *Gray Matters*

PRIVACY

Privacy Background

Privacy in *Privacy and Progress in Whole Genome Sequencing*

Privacy in *Ethics and Ebola: Public Health Planning and Response*

RESEARCH DESIGN

Research Design Background

Research Design in *Gray Matters: Integrative Approaches for Neuroscience, Ethics, and Society*

Research Design in *Ethics and Ebola: Public Health Planning and Response*

VULNERABLE POPULATIONS

Vulnerable Populations Background

Vulnerable Populations in *"Ethically Impossible" STD Research in Guatemala from 1946 to 1948*

Vulnerable Populations in *Safeguarding Children: Pediatric Medical Countermeasure Research*

Vulnerable Populations in *Gray Matters*

User Guides

High School Teachers

Researchers

Human Subjects Researchers

Legal Educators

Public Health Professionals

Public Policy Educators

Science Educators

Webinars

Advancing Bioethics Education

Multidisciplinary Implementation of Bioethics Commission Educational Materials

Ethics and Ebola

Gray Matters: Neuroscience, Ethics, and Society

At the time of printing.

Appendix III: Guest Presenters to the Bioethics Commission Regarding Deliberation and Bioethics Education

Laura Bishop, Ph.D.
Head of Academic Programs
Kennedy Institute of Ethics
Georgetown University

Marion Danis, M.D.
Head, Section on Ethics
and Health Policy
Department of Bioethics
National Institutes of Health
Clinical Center

F. Daniel Davis, Ph.D.
Director of Bioethics
Geisinger Health System

Raymond De Vries, Ph.D.
Professor of Learning Health Sciences
Co-Director, Center for Bioethics
and Social Sciences in Medicine
Professor of Sociology
Professor of Obstetrics and Gynecology
University of Michigan

Florence Evans
Deliberative Poll Participant
What's Next California

James S. Fishkin, Ph.D.
Janet M. Peck Professor of
International Communication
Director, Center for
Deliberative Democracy
Stanford University

John Gastil, Ph.D.
Head and Professor
Communication Arts and Sciences
and Political Science
The Pennsylvania State University

Diana E. Hess, Ph.D.
Professor of Curriculum and Instruction
University of Wisconsin-Madison
Senior Vice President
Spencer Foundation

Sir Roland Jackson
Executive Chair
Sciencewise

Steven Joffe, M.D., M.P.H.
Emanuel and Robert Hart Associate
Professor of Medical Ethics and
Health Policy
Vice Chair for Medical Ethics
Department of Medical Ethics
and Health Policy
Perelman School of Medicine
University of Pennsylvania

Scott Kim, M.D., Ph.D.
Senior Investigator
Department of Bioethics
National Institutes of Health
Clinical Center

Sue Knight, Ph.D.
Curriculum Author
Primary Ethics Limited
Australia

Robert F. Ladenson, Ph.D.
Emeritus Faculty Associate
Center for the Study of Ethics
in the Professions
Illinois Institute of Technology

Lisa M. Lee, Ph.D., M.A., M.S.
Executive Director
Presidential Commission for the
Study of Bioethical Issues

Lisa Lehmann, M.D., Ph.D., M.Sc.
Director, Center for Bioethics
Brigham and Women's Hospital
Associate Professor of Medicine
and Medical Ethics
Harvard Medical School
Associate Professor of Health Policy
and Management
Harvard School of Public Health

Daniel Levin, Ph.D.
Associate Professor
Department of Political Science
University of Utah

Margaret Little, B.Phil., Ph.D.
Director, Kennedy Institute of Ethics
Associate Professor
Philosophy Department
Georgetown University

Seth Mnookin
Associate Director
MIT Graduate Program in
Science Writing

Carol Ripple, Ph.D.
Associate Director for Education
Research and Engagement
Duke University Social Science
Research Institute

Jason L. Schwartz, Ph.D., M. Bioethics
Harold T. Shapiro Fellow in Bioethics
University Center for Human Values
Princeton University

David Steiner, Ph.D.
Executive Director
Johns Hopkins Institute for
Education Policy
Professor, School of Education
Johns Hopkins University

Dennis Thompson, Ph.D.
Alfred North Whitehead Professor of
Political Philosophy
Faculty of Arts and Sciences
Professor of Public Policy
John F. Kennedy School of Government
Harvard University (Emeritus)

Connie Ulrich, Ph.D., R.N., F.A.A.N.
Associate Professor of Bioethics
and Nursing
Department of Biobehavioral
Health Sciences
Secondary Appointment, Department
of Medical Ethics and Health Policy
Associate Director, NewCourtland
Center for Transitions and Health
University of Pennsylvania Schools
of Nursing and Medicine

Presidential Commission for the Study of Bioethical Issues
1425 New York Avenue NW, Suite C-100
Washington, D.C. 20005
(202) 233-3960
http://www.bioethics.gov

www.ingramcontent.com/pod-product-compliance
Lightning Source LLC
Chambersburg PA
CBHW081153180526
45170CB00006B/2054